Food Science
The Biochemistry of Food and Nutrition

Lab Manual
Student Edition

Kay Yockey Mehas
Family and Consumer Sciences Teacher
Principal/Director of Schools
Eugene, Oregon

Sharon Lesley Rodgers
Former Chemistry/Physics Teacher
Henry D. Sheldon High School
Eugene, Oregon

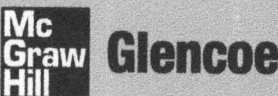

New York, New York   Columbus, Ohio   Chicago, Illinois   Woodland Hills, California

Safety Notice

The reader is expressly advised to consider and use all safety precautions described in this Lab Manual or that might also be indicated by undertaking the activities described herein. In addition, common sense should be exercised to help avoid all potential hazards and, in particular, to take relevant safety precautions concerning any known or likely hazards involved in food preparation, or in use of the procedures described in *Food Science: The Biochemistry of Food and Nutrition*, such as the risk of knife cuts or burns.

Publisher and Authors assume no responsibility for the activities of the reader or for the subject matter experts who prepared this book. Publisher and Author make no representation or warranties of any kind, including but not limited to, the warranties of fitness for particular purpose or merchantability, nor for any implied warranties related thereto, or otherwise. Publisher and Author will not be liable for damages of any type, including any consequential, special or exemplary damages resulting, in whole or in part, from reader's use or reliance upon the information, instructions, warnings or other matter contained in this Lab Manual.

Brand Disclaimer

Publisher does not necessarily recommend or endorse any particular company or brand name product that may be discussed or pictured in this Lab Manual. Brand name products are used because they are readily available, likely to be known to the reader, and their use may aid in the understanding of the Lab Manual. Publisher recognizes that other brand name or generic products may be substituted and work as well or better than those featured in the Lab Manual.

Illustrations: Articulate Graphics

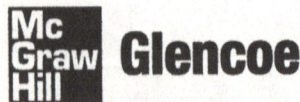

The McGraw-Hill Companies

Copyright © All rights reserved. Except as permitted under the United States Copyright Act, no part of this publication may be reproduced or distributed in any form or by any means, or stored in a database or retrieval system, without prior written permission of the publisher, Glencoe/McGraw-Hill.

Send all inquiries to:
Glencoe/McGraw-Hill
21600 Oxnard St., Suite 500
Woodland Hills, CA 91367

ISBN 0-07-869082-X

Printed in the United States of America

8 9 10 11 12 LHN 25 24 23 22

Table of Contents

The Food Science Lab

Using the Lab Manual...7
Metric Reference Charts..9
Sample Lab Report Form..10

Working Safely in the Lab

Basic Lab Safety Rules...11
Safety Symbols in Food Science...12
    Personal Hygiene Safety Guidelines..12
    Chemical Safety Guidelines...13
    Electrical Safety Guidelines...13
    Sharp Object Safety Guidelines...14
    Eye Safety Guidelines..14
    Fire Safety Guidelines..15
    Hand Safety Guidelines...15
    Clothing Safety Guidelines..16
    Equipment Safety Guidelines..16
    Proper Waste Disposal Guidelines..16
Safety Awareness Checklist..17
First Aid in the Lab...20
Lab Safety Agreement...21

Understanding Lab Techniques

Working with Chemicals..22
Measuring Temperature and Volume..24
Measuring Mass with the Electronic Balance..25
Measuring Mass with the Triple-Beam Balance..26
Lighting a Laboratory Burner...28
Using a Microscope...29
Inserting Glass Tubing into a Rubber Stopper..30
Using a Buret...31
Filtering Substances..32

Building Skills

Using the Scientific Method...33
Evaluating Laboratory Situations...35
Estimating Metric Measurements..39
Creating Line Graphs..43
Creating Tables...45
Creating Bar Graphs...47
Creating Pie Charts...49

Conducting Lab Experiments

Unit 1
2-1 Food Labels and Nutrition 51
2-2 Packaged Food Scavenger Hunt 53

Unit 2
3-1 Using an Electronic Balance 55
3-2 Precision in Measurement 57
4-1 Measuring the Volume of a Liquid 59
4-2 Using a Graduated Cylinder 61
4-3 Mass and Volume of Beans 63
5-1 Properties of Popping Corn 67
6-1 Odor Recognition 69
6-2 Flavor Comparison 71
6-3 Mouthfeel and Sensory Evaluation 73

Unit 3
7-1 Separating Mixtures 75
7-2 Heterogeneous and Homogeneous Mixtures 77
7-3 The Boiling Point of Water 79
8-1 Physical Changes and Chemical Reactions 81
8-2 Changes Involved in Making Peanut Brittle 85
8-3 Boiling Points of Sugar and Salt Solutions 87
9-1 The Solvent Properties of Water 89
9-2 Purifying Water 91
9-3 Bottled Water Taste Test 93
10-1 Neutralization 95
10-2 The pH of Common Foods 97
10-3 Red Cabbage Juice Indicator 99
11-1 Effect of Surface Area on Cooking Rate 101
11-2 Effect of Temperature on Cooking Rate 103
11-3 Heat Transfer Through Metal 105

Unit 4
12-1 Identifying Basic Nutrients in Foods 107
12-2 Calcium in Milk 111
12-3 Nutrition Facts Panel 113
13-1 Digestion of Starch 117
13-2 Osmosis 119
14-1 Kcalories in Food 123
14-2 Cellular Respiration 125
15-1 Thickening Agents 127
15-2 Making Fondant 131
16-1 Effect of Light on Flavor 135
16-2 Fat Content of Beef 137

16-3 Lipids and Tenderizing 139
17-1 The Effect of Acid on Protein 141
17-2 Egg Foam Stability 143
18-1 Iron as an Additive in Cereals 145
18-2 Titration of Vitamin C 147

Unit 5

19-1 Enzymes in Foods 151
19-2 Enzymatic Browning 153
19-3 Effect of Blanching on Enzymes 155
20-1 Temperature and Solubility 157
20-2 Making an Emulsion 161
20-3 Sensory Evaluation of Gelatin Dessert 163
21-1 Using Baking Powders to Produce Carbon Dioxide 165
21-2 Comparison of Leavening Agents 167
22-1 Yeast Growth 171
22-2 Fermentation of Pickles 173
22-3 Lactic-Acid Fermentation 175
23-1 Separating Milk 177
23-2 Making Yogurt 179
23-3 Evaluation of Commercial Yogurts 181
24-1 Testing for Food Additives 183
24-2 Pudding Mixes and Additives 185
24-3 Effects of Minerals on Protein 189

Unit 6

25-1 Growing Cultures 193
25-2 Bacteria in Milk 195
26-1 Dehydrating Beef 197
26-2 Dehydrating Fruits and Vegetables 199
26-3 Reconstituting Fruits and Vegetables 201
27-1 Evaluating Canned Peas 203
27-2 Environment and Bacteria 205
28-1 Orange Juice Comparison 207

Using the Lab Manual

As a student of food science, you'll read how chemistry principles apply to food. This information has been gathered and researched by scientists for many years. Chemistry, however, is much more than just reading about scientific principles. It's also conducting experiments yourself to see what happens firsthand and to even make discoveries of your own. Experimentation in the food science lab will be a major part of your study, and this lab manual will be your guide.

Safety Concerns

The early pages in the Lab Manual include safety guidelines. As you prepare for lab work, be sure to read these pages carefully. Reading and understanding the guidelines will help you work correctly and responsibly with chemicals and lab equipment in order to protect yourself and those around you.

Also, be sure you are familiar with first-aid procedures. A chart that shows some basic responses is on page 20. Once you are familiar with the safety expectations and first-aid procedures, you should sign the Lab Safety Agreement on page 21.

Other Manual Contents

Your manual also contains tips on how to perform certain lab techniques and use equipment. You'll learn how to work with chemicals, light a lab burner, and a number of other techniques.

To help prepare you for effective lab work and the creation of informative lab reports, several skill-building exercises are also provided in this manual. These activities are listed in the table of contents, along with all other components of the manual.

Lab Experiments

The largest part of this manual is the set of lab experiments. A quick scan of these pages will introduce you to the interesting explorations ahead. The experiments, which have a consistent format that will eventually become quite familiar to you, are described below.

- **Safety First.** At the top of each experiment are symbols that draw attention to specific safety requirements. All symbols and guidelines are explained on pages 12-16 in this manual. Before you begin each experiment, fill in the appropriate line of the checklist on pages 17-19. Doing so will indicate to your teacher that you are aware of the specific safety rules that apply to the experiment you're about to perform.
- **Introduction.** A short opener tells you about each experiment. Any needed background information is provided, along with a statement about the objective.
- **Equipment and Materials.** This portion of each experiment lists the equipment and materials you need. Gather them before you start, following any special instructions from your teacher about securing chemicals.
- **Procedure.** The numbered steps in the procedure tell you how to carry out each experiment. Before you begin, read all steps fully. If you're assigned to one variation within an experiment, do only that part. Measuring correctly, following teacher instructions, and completing the procedure carefully will help you get accurate results.
- **Analyzing Results.** When you answer the questions in this section, you examine and comment on what occurred in the experiment. You may be asked to apply observations to other situations.
- **Data Table.** Throughout each procedure, you will be asked to record data in a table. For some experiments, you will transfer your findings onto the board and then add the data from other groups to your table. Occasionally, you may need to expand the data table on your own paper to compile a complete set of classroom results.

During and after an experiment, a lab report should be completed. Your teacher will provide you with a form, or you can create one based on the sample shown on page 10 in this manual. Any conclusions you reach will be reported on this form.

A Positive Experience

Most students enjoy their work in the food science lab. Seeing scientific principles in action brings a sense of discovery and heightens understanding. For some students, lab work even inspires them to explore the possibility of a career in food science. Whatever your aim, you'll come away with new skills and awareness as you work cooperatively and seriously with others in the food science lab.

Metric Reference Charts

Common Metric Units

	Metric Unit	English Equivalent
Length	1 centimeter (cm) = 10 millimeters (mm) 100 centimeters = 1 meter (m)	1 cm = 2.5 in. 1 m = 40 in.
Mass	1 gram (g) = 1000 milligrams (mg) 1000 grams = 1 kilogram (kg)	1 g = 0.036 oz. 1 kg = 2.2 lbs.
Volume	1 liter (L) = 1000 milliliters (mL)	1 L = 1 qt. = 4 c.

Metric Conversion Chart

	When you want to convert:	Multiply by:	To find:
Length	inches centimeters feet meters yards meters miles kilometers	2.54 0.39 0.30 3.28 0.91 1.09 1.61 0.62	centimeters inches meters feet meters yards kilometers miles
Volume	cubic inches cubic centimeters cubic feet cubic meters liters liters gallons	16.39 0.06 0.03 35.31 1.06 0.26 3.78	cubic centimeters cubic inches cubic meters cubic feet quarts gallons liters
Mass	ounces grams pounds kilograms	28.35 0.04 0.45 2.20	grams ounces kilograms pounds

Converting Temperatures

Fahrenheit to Celsius	°C = 5/9 (°F − 32)
Celsius to Fahrenheit	°F = 9/5 (°C + 32)

Food Science Lab Manual
Copyright © Mehas & Rodgers

Sample Lab Report Form

(Before conducting the experiment, fill in everything down to "Results." During and after the experiment, complete the rest.)

Number and Title of Experiment: _1-A: Using a Triple-Beam Balance_

Performed By: _(your name)_ **Class:** _4_

Partner: _(your partner's name)_ **Date:** _September 6_

Purpose
To become familiar with the triple-beam balance.

Procedure
Check the balance for accuracy when the pan is empty. Place objects on the pan and adjust weights. Read the mass indicated. Record the mass of the object in your data table.

Results

Observations: _The mass of the scissors was the greatest._
The triple-beam balance was hard to adjust.

Data:

Object	Mass
Paper clip	5.0 g
Beaker	126.8 g
Scissors	196.9 g

Calculations: _This example uses weighing paper._
Mass of weighing paper was 4.0 g.
Mass of paper and paper clip was 9.0 g.
Subtract mass of weighing paper from total mass.
9.0 g – 4.0 g = mass of paper clip.

Analyzing Results:
1. _The mass of a penny would be closer to 1.0 g._
2. _Mass an empty 10-mL graduated cylinder, add exactly 10 mL of water, and mass again. The mass of the water is the difference between the two readings._

Conclusion
When accuracy is important in measuring mass, the triple-beam balance should be used. The triple-beam balance can be time-consuming to use, but it is very accurate.

Basic Lab Safety Rules

Working in the food science lab can be an interesting and rewarding part of this course. The lab is still a classroom, however. Take your work seriously. You will promote not only learning, but safety as well. Following the rules listed here will help make lab work a safe and useful experience for everyone.

When conducting an experiment...

1. Study the procedure before you come to the lab. Read all directions several times. Be sure you understand any safety symbols shown on the page.
2. Follow the steps exactly as written. Pay close attention to additional oral instructions and demonstrations given by your teacher. If you have questions about any aspect of the procedure, ask your teacher for an explanation.
3. Obtain your teacher's permission before trying an activity not included in the experiment.
4. Stay at your assigned location as much as possible. Minimize noise and other disruptions that could affect concentration and lead to accident or injury.
5. Keep lanes to exits clear of clutter and activity.
6. Do not bring food or beverages into the lab.
7. Use safety equipment as instructed.
8. Report any accident or injury, even a minor one, to your teacher.
9. Clean up any spills immediately. Dilute solutions with water before removing.
10. Know the location and proper use of the first-aid kit.
11. Know the location of the school nurse's office.
12. Obtain your teacher's permission to enter the lab outside of class time, and work only when a teacher is present.
13. Never work alone.

After conducting an experiment...

1. Check that water and gas are off. Disconnect electrical equipment.
2. Carefully wash materials and equipment as instructed.
3. Return all materials to their proper place.
4. Clean your work area before leaving the lab.

Safety Symbols in Food Science

As you advance in this course, you'll learn that symbols are a popular form of shorthand for food scientists. Among the most important symbols you'll encounter in your lab manual are the ones for lab safety. You'll find them at the top of most experiments. These alert you to the need for safe practices and remind you of possible hazards associated with each lab procedure. The chart below shows the safety symbols and summarizes their meaning. On the pages that follow, you'll find more detailed explanations of these symbols.

Safety Symbols for Food Scientists

🚿	**Personal Hygiene.** Safe personal habits are especially important in the experiment.	🔥	**Fire Safety.** The procedure requires use of a burner or other heat source.
☠	**Chemical Safety.** Substances used in the experiment require special handling and precautions.	🧤	**Hand Safety.** Some steps in the experiment call for particular attention to hand safety.
⚡	**Electrical Safety.** The procedure requires use of electrical equipment and electrical safety practices.	👕	**Clothing Safety.** Take precautions to protect your clothing during the experiment.
☝	**Sharp Object Safety.** The experiment uses lab glassware; take needed precautions.	🥤	**Equipment Safety.** The experiment requires proper use and care of specialized lab equipment.
🥽	**Eye Safety.** Some conditions of the experiment require special attention to eye safety.	🗑	**Proper Waste Disposal.** Waste or chemicals used in the experiment require appropriate disposal.

Personal Hygiene

This symbol serves as a reminder for safe personal habits in the lab. Follow the guidelines below when you see this symbol.

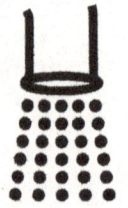

1. Wash hands with soap and water before beginning labs. This is especially important if you will create or sample food products.
2. Handle microorganisms grown in a petri dish or test tube with care. Use correct sterile techniques when transferring to a microscope slide or from one culture to another.
3. Avoid touching your face or mouth with your hands.
4. Wash hands thoroughly after handling chemicals or containers that hold them.
5. Wash your hands thoroughly after cleanup.

12   **Food Science Lab Manual**
Copyright © Mehas & Rodgers

Chemical Safety

The chemical safety symbol alerts you that substances used in the experiment require special handling and precautions. Follow the guidelines below when you see this symbol.

When preparing for an experiment . . .
1. Wear safety goggles if working with dangerous chemicals that could spill or any chemicals that could spatter. Your teacher will indicate when goggles are needed.
2. Take chemicals from labeled containers only. Check with your teacher if you have any questions about the label on a container.
3. Read labels on chemical containers and reagent bottles twice before using. Double-check them against the instructions to be sure you have the ones needed.
4. Follow any specific instructions provided by your teacher for using a particular chemical.
5. Keep the container lid closed when a chemical is not in use.

When conducting an experiment...
1. Use the exact amount of a chemical called for.
2. Complete your data table promptly as a running record of the chemicals you have used in a procedure.
3. Do not taste any substance unless instructed as part of the procedure.
4. Mix chemicals only when, and as, instructed.
5. Keep your hands away from your face and mouth, and wash your hands before leaving the lab.
6. Don't eat or drink from lab glassware.
7. Thoroughly wash and dry a container used for a chemical before placing a different chemical in it.
8. Keep your science drawer locked when not in use to ensure that the equipment is used only by food science classes for food science labs.
9. Always return chemical materials to the teacher for proper storage at the end of the lab.

In case of accident...
1. Report chemical spills to the teacher.
2. Avoid contact of skin and clothing with acids and bases. If contact occurs, rinse immediately with cool water and alert the teacher.
3. If a mercury thermometer breaks, notify your teacher immediately for proper disposal. Do not touch the mercury.

Electrical Safety

This symbol alerts you that the procedure requires use of electrical equipment and electrical safety practices. Follow the guidelines below when you see this symbol.

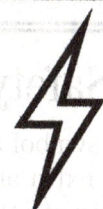

1. Do not use equipment with frayed cords, loose connections, or exposed wires. Immediately report such damage to your teacher.
2. Be sure electrical equipment is grounded properly.
3. Handle electrical equipment with dry hands only.
4. Since the human body is a conductor of electricity, leave one hand free, not touching anything, when plugging or unplugging an electrical appliance.
5. Always unplug electrical equipment by grasping the plug, not the cord. Unplug from the wall before detaching from the appliance.

Food Science Lab Manual
Copyright © Mehas & Rodgers

6. Keep cords and electrical appliances a safe distance from heat sources and sinks, where they could be damaged or create a hazard.
7. Place electrical cords away from traffic zones where someone could trip on them.
8. Keep work areas dry, including floors and countertops.
9. Never overload an electric circuit.
10. Turn off and unplug unattended electrical equipment. Store properly before leaving the lab.

Sharp Object Safety

This symbol reminds you to take precautions when using lab glassware. Follow the guidelines below when you see this symbol.

1. Do not use broken, chipped, or cracked glassware; alert your teacher of broken items.
2. Air-dry glassware when possible.
3. If glassware breaks, make sure it is cool before picking it up. Use a damp paper towel, never your bare hands.
4. Place glassware away from edges of work surfaces, where it could fall or be tipped over.
5. Use an insulating pad beneath hot glassware when setting it on a countertop.
6. Use only heat-resistant glassware to heat or store hot materials.
7. Place a wire gauze between the glass and the flame when heating flasks and beakers. Don't heat graduated cylinders over a burner.
8. Never use a thermometer to stir a liquid.

Eye Safety

This symbol alerts you that some conditions of the experiment require extra attention to eye safety. Follow the guidelines below when you see this symbol.

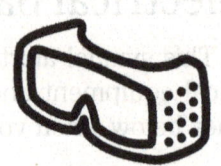

1. Wear approved safety goggles in the lab when heating substances or working with certain chemicals and when instructed by your teacher or the experiment directions.
2. Know the location of the emergency eye-wash station and how to use the eye-wash equipment.
3. Never heat a liquid in a closed container; the expanding gases could cause glass to shatter.
4. Avoid wearing contact lenses, if possible. They absorb vapors, even under safety goggles, and can be hard to remove in an emergency.

Fire Safety

This symbol alerts you that the procedure involves the use of a burner or other heat source. Follow the guidelines below when you see this symbol.

1. Notify lab partners when igniting a burner in the lab.
2. Never reach across an open flame.
3. Turn off burners when not in use.
4. Keep potholders and cloth or paper towels away from open flames.
5. Do not heat substances unless specified in the lab. Some generally safe chemicals become hazardous when heated.
6. Bring objects or substances into contact with a flame only when told to do so.
7. Never use an open flame if working with volatile liquids, such as alcohol.
8. Never leave unattended any substance that is being heated or visibly reacting.
9. Dispose of used matches properly as directed by your teacher; never throw them into a wastepaper basket.
10. Take only required books and papers into the lab; keep them a safe distance from burners.
11. Know the location and proper use of the fire alarm, fire extinguisher, fire blanket, and safety shower. Be familiar with fire exits and fire drill procedures.
12. If a fire breaks out, or if your clothing catches fire, smother the flames with the fire blanket or a coat, or get under a safety shower. *Never run.*

Hand Safety

This symbol tells you that some steps in the experiment call for particular attention to hand safety. Follow the guidelines below when you see this symbol.

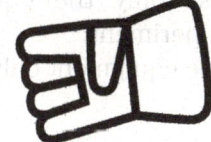

1. Wear gloves or use a cloth to protect hands when inserting thermometers in rubber stoppers.
2. Check glassware for heat before picking up; hot glassware looks the same as cool.
3. Use thoroughly dry potholders to avoid heat transfer that could cause a burn.
4. Use appropriate tongs for handling hot containers. When possible, allow heated materials time to cool before handling.
5. Use knives only for their intended purpose.
6. Carry knives and other sharp utensils in clean, dry hands, with the point turned down and away from you and others.
7. Cut away from your body when slicing foods.
8. Don't try to catch a knife as it falls.
9. Don't use knives to point or gesture.
10. Store knives so they are easy to distinguish and pick up.
11. Never use a cutting device with more than one edge.

Food Science Lab Manual
Copyright © Mehas & Rodgers

Clothing Safety

This symbol reminds you to take certain precautions to protect yourself and your clothing while working in the lab. Follow the guidelines below when you see this symbol.

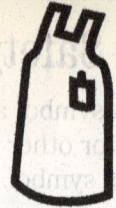

1. Wear a lab apron while conducting an experiment.
2. Remove a jacket before beginning a lab.
3. Wear footwear that provides full foot protection.
4. Remove dangling jewelry.
5. Tie back long hair and loose clothing.

Equipment Safety

This symbol reminds you of general rules for using the specialized equipment of a lab. Follow the guidelines below when you see this symbol.

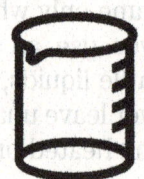

1. Be sure you know how to use a piece of equipment before starting a lab; otherwise ask for help.
2. Use only the equipment required in an experiment.
3. Use equipment only for its intended purpose.
4. Observe safety precautions related to each specific piece of equipment.
5. Transport equipment carefully and with proper support.
6. Return equipment to its proper location after use.

Proper Waste Disposal

This symbol refers to appropriate disposal of waste or chemicals. Follow the guidelines below when you see this symbol.

1. Follow your teacher's instruction for waste disposal, especially for chemical and microbial materials.
2. Place broken glass and solid substances in the proper containers. Never discard materials in the sink.
3. Place paper toweling and other disposable cleaning supplies in the wastepaper basket.

Safety Awareness Checklist

Directions: After reading each assigned lab experiment, check the safety concerns that apply. This must be completed and approved before you begin each experiment.

Experiment	Safety Awareness Symbols									
2-1 Food Labels and Nutrition										
2-2 Packaged Food Scavenger Hunt										
3-1 Using an Electronic Balance										
3-2 Precision in Measurement										
4-1 Measuring the Volume of a Liquid										
4-2 Using a Graduated Cylinder										
4-3 Mass and Volume of Beans										
5-1 Properties of Popping Corn										
6-1 Odor Recognition										
6-2 Flavor Comparison										
6-3 Mouthfeel and Sensory Evaluation										
7-1 Separating Mixtures										
7-2 Heterogeneous and Homogeneous Mixtures										
7-3 The Boiling Point of Water										
8-1 Physical Changes and Chemical Reactions										
8-2 Changes Involved in Making Peanut Brittle										
8-3 Boiling Points of Sugar and Salt Solutions										
9-1 The Solvent Properties of Water										
9-2 Purifying Water										

Food Science Lab Manual
Copyright © Mehas & Rodgers

Experiment	Safety Awareness Symbols									
	🚿	☠	⚡	☞	👓	🔥	🧤	🧴	🥫	🗑
9-3 Bottled Water Taste Test										
10-1 Neutralization										
10-2 The pH of Common Foods										
10-3 Red Cabbage Juice Indicator										
11-1 Effect of Surface Area on Cooking Rate										
11-2 Effect of Temperature on Cooking Rate										
11-3 Heat Transfer Through Metal										
12-1 Identifying Basic Nutrients in Foods										
12-2 Calcium in Milk										
12-3 Nutrition Facts Panel										
13-1 Digestion of Starch										
13-2 Osmosis										
14-1 Kcalories in Food										
14-2 Cellular Respiration										
15-1 Thickening Agents										
15-2 Making Fondant										
16-1 Effect of Light on Flavor										
16-2 Fat Content of Beef										
16-3 Lipids and Tenderizing										
17-1 The Effect of Acid on Protein										
17-2 Egg Foam Stability										
18-1 Iron as an Additive in Cereals										
18-2 Titration of Vitamin C										
19-1 Enzymes in Foods										
19-2 Enzymatic Browning										

Experiment	Safety Awareness Symbols								
19-3 Effect of Blanching on Enzymes									
20-1 Temperature and Solubility									
20-2 Making an Emulsion									
20-3 Sensory Evaluation of Gelatin Dessert									
21-1 Using Baking Powders to Produce Carbon Dioxide									
21-2 Comparison of Leavening Agents									
22-1 Yeast Growth									
22-2 Fermentation of Pickles									
22-3 Lactic-Acid Fermentation									
23-1 Separating Milk									
23-2 Making Yogurt									
23-3 Evaluation of Commercial Yogurts									
24-1 Testing for Food Additives									
24-2 Pudding Mixes and Additives									
24-3 Effects of Minerals on Protein									
25-1 Growing Cultures									
25-2 Bacteria in Milk									
26-1 Dehydrating Beef									
26-2 Dehydrating Fruits and Vegetables									
26-3 Reconstituting Fruits and Vegetables									
27-1 Evaluating Canned Peas									
27-2 Environment and Bacteria									
28-1 Orange Juice Comparison									

Food Science Lab Manual
Copyright © Mehas & Rodgers

First Aid in the Lab

Alertness and a good safety policy are solid defenses against accidents. Whenever you work with chemicals, burners, and sharp objects, however, injuries are possible. Then, your best allies are a cool head, a well-stocked first-aid kit, and a quick and appropriate response. The chart below briefly outlines safe responses to injuries you may encounter in the food science lab.

Remember that first aid is immediate care only. All injuries, even minor ones, should be reported to your teacher and to the school nurse, since further medical attention may be needed. If a school nurse is not available, assistance may be needed from other emergency medical professionals. Call immediately for professional help in the event of any serious injury.

Injury	Response	Notes
Thermal (heat) burns	Bathe area generously with cold water; immerse, if possible, until cool. If school health care provider is not available, clean with soap and water. Apply antibiotic ointment and dry, sterile dressing.	Do not remove clothing that sticks to the skin.
Chemical burns	Remove contaminated clothing if possible. Flush with plenty of cold water until medical help arrives. If school health care provider is not available, flush injury with water and apply boric acid to base burns and baking soda to acid burns. If eye is affected, flush outward from nasal passages.	If treating another person, protect yourself from contact with the chemical.
Electrical burns	Look for both entry and exit burns. Cover burns with a dry, sterile dressing; do not apply water.	Electrical shock can stop the heart; watch for such signs as shortness of breath and chest pains.
Cuts	Cover wound with sterile dressing. Raise injured area above the heart. Apply direct pressure for at least 5 minutes. For serious injuries, seek emergency help. For minor injuries, if school health professional is not available, clean wound with soap and water, removing foreign matter. Dress with antibiotic ointment and sterile dressing.	If treating another person, wear gloves to avoid contact with blood; wash hands thoroughly afterwards.
Fainting	Have person lie down with legs raised about eight inches. Loosen restrictive clothing.	Check for injury caused by falling.
Poisoning	Determine cause of poisoning. Call the nearest poison control center; be ready with information about the person and poison.	Induce vomiting only if instructed; some poisons damage the mouth and esophagus during vomiting.

Lab Safety Agreement

My signature on this form indicates that I have carefully read all of the safety rules for working in the Food Science Lab. I am aware of my responsibility in keeping the work environment safe. I also recognize the importance of the following:

- Reading directions thoroughly before beginning an activity.
- Following instructions during a procedure.
- Protecting eyes, face, hands, and body while conducting activities.
- Understanding first-aid procedures.
- Knowing the use and location of first-aid and fire-fighting equipment.
- Conducting myself responsibly in the lab at all times.

I agree to abide by the regulations and procedures associated with the above concerns as well as any additional instructions provided by my teacher or the school district during the school year.

Signed: _____

Class: _____

Date: _____

Food Science Lab Manual
Copyright © Mehas & Rodgers

Working with Chemicals

Technically, all the substances you use in the food science lab are chemicals. However, some substances are of more concern than others. Some can be irritating and even hazardous if not handled correctly.

To prepare for an experiment, you'll obtain the chemicals you need from stock bottles provided by your teacher. You will transfer the chemicals to your containers and then perhaps transfer them again as you complete an experiment. When working with chemicals, remember that you should *never touch chemicals with your hands*. Also, always wear safety goggles and a protective apron when using chemicals that your teacher tells you are hazardous.

The guidelines that follow explain some general principles and procedures related to your work with chemicals. Follow them carefully to promote safe and successful lab results.

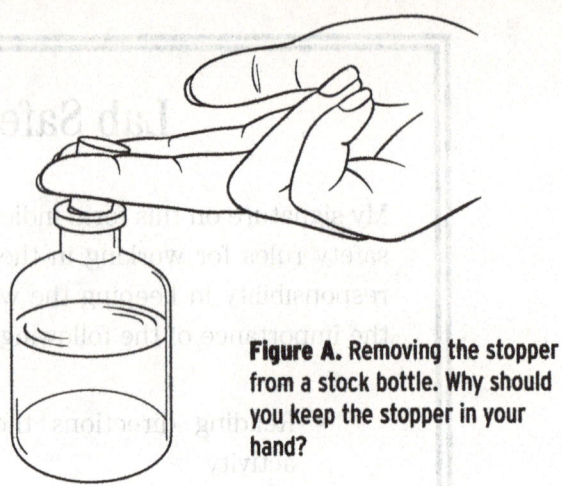

Figure A. Removing the stopper from a stock bottle. Why should you keep the stopper in your hand?

Obtaining Chemicals for an Experiment

- When obtaining chemicals for an experiment, leave stock bottles in the location specified by your teacher. Carry a small amount of the needed substance to your work area in an appropriate container.
- Take only the amount of chemical needed. Unused amounts cannot be returned to the bottle because the rest of the stock might become contaminated.
- If you are gathering multiple chemicals that look similar, mark the containers or massing paper with the name of the substance.

Transferring Liquid Chemicals

1. To open a stock bottle, grasp the stopper between your fingers (**Figure A**) and remove it from the bottle. Hold the stopper until you're ready to close the bottle; to prevent possible contamination, don't set the stopper on any surface.
2. As you pour, stand over a sink to catch spills. Hold the container at eye level.
3. Pour the chemical from the bottle until you have the amount needed, reading the volume marked on the container. Use only this process; don't dip a dropper into the stock bottle since this also risks contamination.
4. Replace the stopper in the reagent bottle.
5. If any liquid runs down the outside of the bottle, rinse it with water before returning it to the shelf. Wipe the bottle with a damp paper towel if the liquid is an acid.
6. To transfer the liquid chemicals again between other containers, use a dropper or other suction bulb.

Transferring Solids

1. Solid chemicals are usually stored in wide-mouth bottles. Remove the substance with a clean spoon or spatula (**Figure B**). As an alternative, carefully shake out the substance by rotating the bottle.

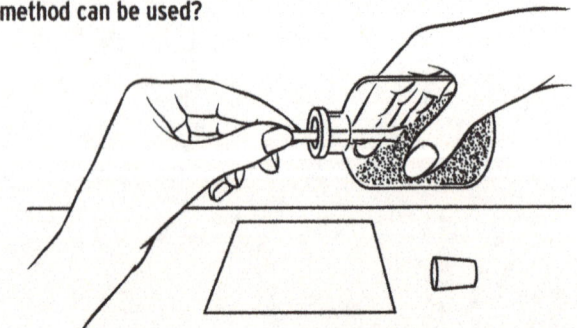

Figure B. Removing a solid from a stock bottle. What other method can be used?

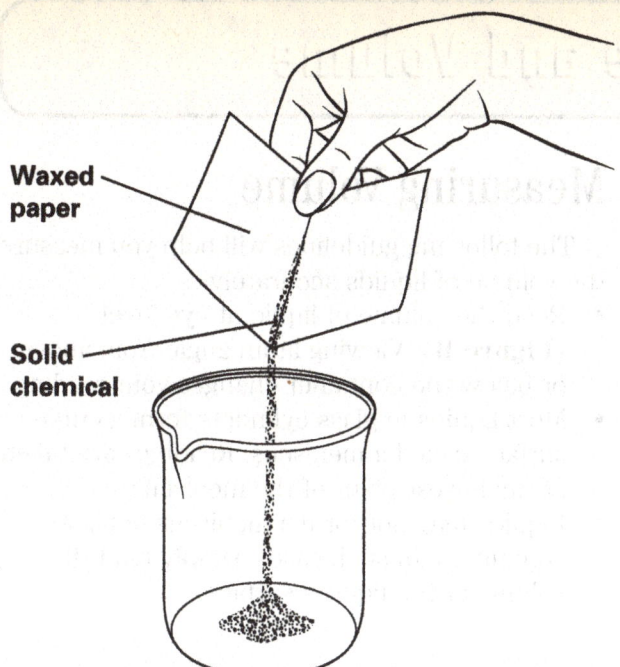

Figure C. Transferring a solid. What purpose does the crease in the paper serve?

2. Dispense the solid onto a piece of creased waxed or massing paper. Using the crease as a channel, slide the solid into the container (**Figure C**). If the solid is going into a test tube, you can roll the waxed paper into a cylinder that fits into the top of the tube. This helps you contain some solids better. Roll the paper with the solid on it carefully as you slip the paper into the test tube (**Figure D**).
3. If the solid is to be massed, remember to use a paper or container. Don't place the chemical directly on the balance pan.

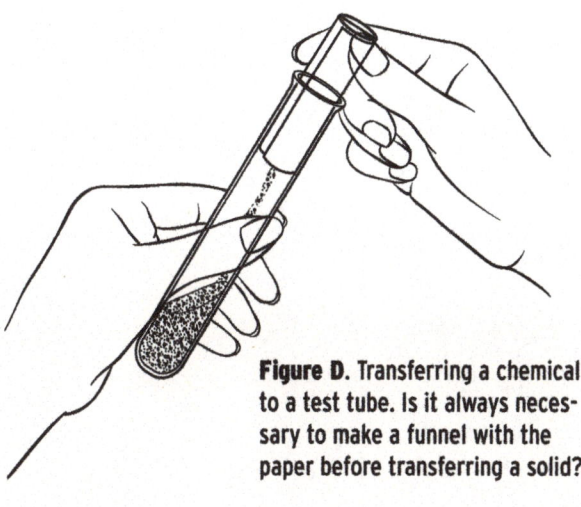

Figure D. Transferring a chemical to a test tube. Is it always necessary to make a funnel with the paper before transferring a solid?

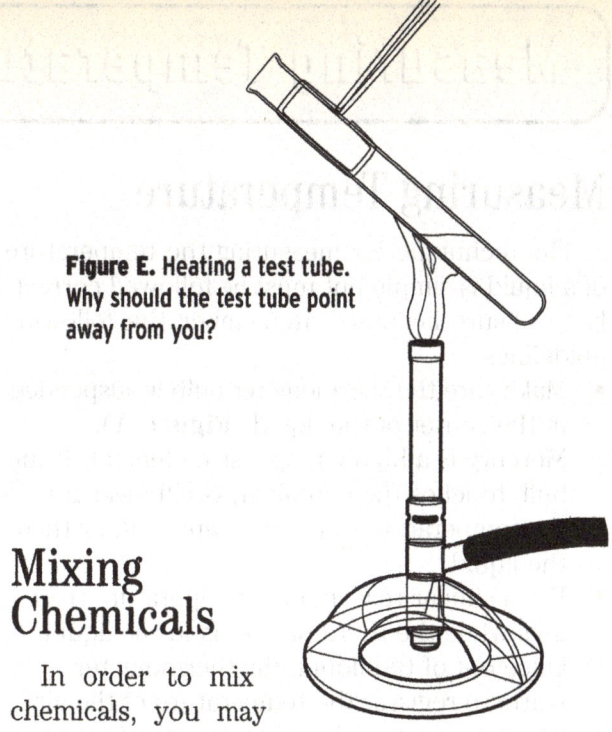

Figure E. Heating a test tube. Why should the test tube point away from you?

Mixing Chemicals

In order to mix chemicals, you may need to shake a test tube gently or heat the substances. Always point the test tube away from yourself and others (**Figure E**). Never look directly into the tube. When heating, move the test tube constantly to heat evenly.

Checking the Aroma of a Chemical Mixture

To check the aroma of a chemical mixture, fan the air above the substance to direct the vapor toward you (**Figure F**). Sniff carefully, without directly inhaling the fumes.

Learning to measure temperature and volume properly is essential to carrying out food science experiments successfully.

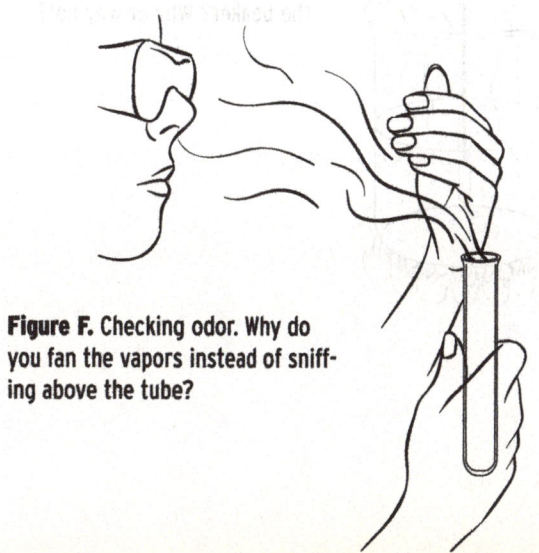

Figure F. Checking odor. Why do you fan the vapors instead of sniffing above the tube?

Measuring Temperature and Volume

Measuring Temperature

The technique for measuring the temperature of a liquid is simple but must be followed correctly to ensure accuracy. Remember the following guidelines:
- Make sure the thermometer bulb is suspended in the center of the liquid (**Figure A**). Mercury is a highly responsive element. If the bulb touches the container, you'll measure the temperature of the container rather than the liquid.
- For a similar reason, take temperature readings while the thermometer is in the liquid. Once out of the liquid, the thermometer starts to register the temperature of the air.
- When measuring the temperature of very hot or boiling liquids, be sure the thermometer you use is calibrated to that temperature range.
- Laboratory thermometers are not designed to be shaken down, as some medical thermometers are. Therefore, do not try to do so.

Measuring Volume

The following guidelines will help you measure the volume of liquids accurately:
- Read the volume of liquid at eye level (**Figure B**). Viewing at an angle from above or below the container changes your reading.
- Most liquids in glass cylinders form a curved surface called a meniscus. Readings are taken at the lowest point of the meniscus.
- Liquids may not form a meniscus in plastic containers. In such cases, simply read the volume at the liquid's surface.

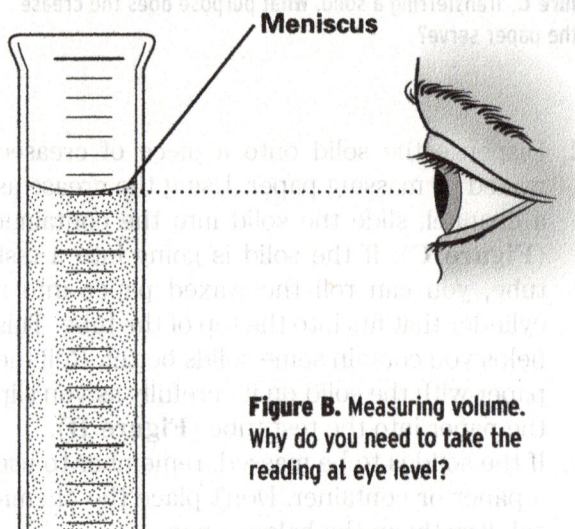

Figure B. Measuring volume. Why do you need to take the reading at eye level?

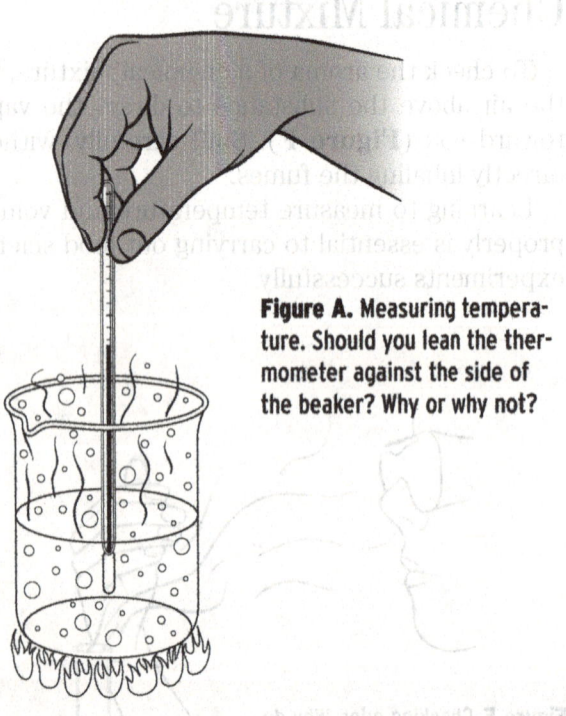

Figure A. Measuring temperature. Should you lean the thermometer against the side of the beaker? Why or why not?

Measuring Mass with the Electronic Balance

The electronic balance is a sensitive instrument capable of measuring remarkably small masses. This is a real advantage for dealing with the tiny amounts of substances often used in the food science lab. You'll want to use the electronic balance properly to help ensure correct results and avoid damage to the equipment.

An electronic balance has a pan on the top where materials to be massed are placed (**Figure A**). Some materials can be massed directly on the pan —solid objects, for example. To protect the balance from caustic substances and to hold materials that spread, however, you'll need a container. Chemical substances must be placed in a container or on massing paper. Use glass or plastic containers for liquid chemicals, and glass or plastic containers or massing paper for solid substances.

Due to air currents caused by heat, a hot object placed directly on the balance pan may give an incorrect value. You'll avoid this problem by letting a heated substance cool before massing.

On the front of an electronic balance are two buttons. One is marked "tare" and the other, "function." Do *not* press the function button unless instructed to do so by your teacher, since this will change the unit of measurement. Pushing the tare button reduces the readout to 0.00 g regardless of what has already been placed on the pan. Use the tare button as you follow one of the procedures for massing.

Massing without a Container

1. Push the tare button so that the digital display reads 0.00 g.
2. Place the item on the balance pan and read the value shown on the screen.

Massing with a Container

If the mass of the container is not needed for your calculations . . .

1. Set the container on the pan and press the tare button. This cancels the container mass, returning the reading to 0.00 g. (Do this step even for massing paper.)
2. Add the substance to be massed to the container. The balance will record the value for the substance alone.

If the mass of the container is needed for your calculations . . .

1. Press the tare button to return the readout to 0.00 g.
2. Place the empty container on the balance pan and record that value.
3. Add the substance and record the combined value.
4. Subtract the container mass from the total to find the mass of the substance itself.

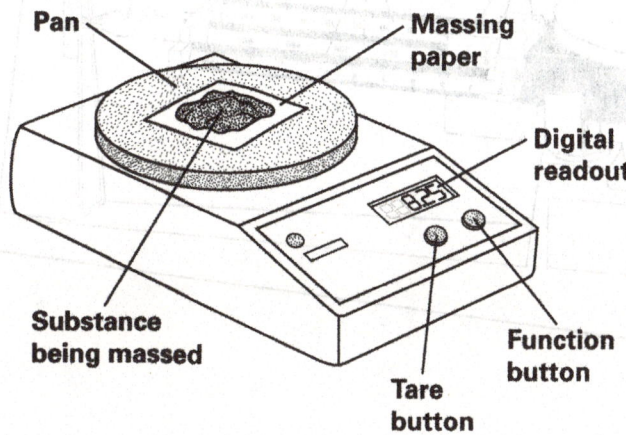

Figure A. The electronic balance you use may be similar to the one shown here. Why must you avoid pressing the function button?

Food Science Lab Manual
Copyright © Mehas & Rodgers

Measuring Mass with the Triple-Beam Balance

As its name implies, the triple-beam balance works on the principle of balance. It measures mass by balancing the object or substance in the pan with weights, or riders, that move along the beams.

Triple-beam balances come in different designs. Although most have three beams, you will find some models with four. The combined value of the riders equals the mass of the item in the pan. When using the balance, you can determine the mass of a substance, or you can set the riders first and then subtract or add to the substance to get the amount you need.

All triple-beam balances have the parts shown in **Figure A**, and all require the same care and technique to yield correct readings.

Transporting the Balance

If you must carry a triple-beam balance to and from your lab station, do so carefully. Follow the steps below to prevent damage.
1. Make sure all riders are set at the zero point.
2. If the pan has a lock mechanism, be sure it is on.
3. Carry the balance with one hand underneath it and the other on the vertical bar that supports the beams.

Preparing the Balance

To prepare a triple-beam balance, you must do a form of calibration. This routine, which is described below, helps ensure reliable results.
1. Slide all riders to the zero point.
2. Check the swing of the pointer. You'll notice that it swings through a set of lines with a midpoint. If the pointer stops, it must stop on the midpoint to be calibrated correctly. You need not wait until the pointer stops, however; just be sure it is swinging an equal distance above and below the midpoint.
3. Turn the adjustment screw, if needed, until the swing of the pointer is correct.

Using the Balance

Measuring mass with a triple-beam balance takes a bit of skill and attention. As with an electronic balance, a container must be used to mass chemicals and hot objects on a triple-beam balance. Note, too that the triple-beam balance has no tare feature. To find the mass of a substance, you need to record the mass of the empty container first and then subtract that value from the mass of the container and substance together.

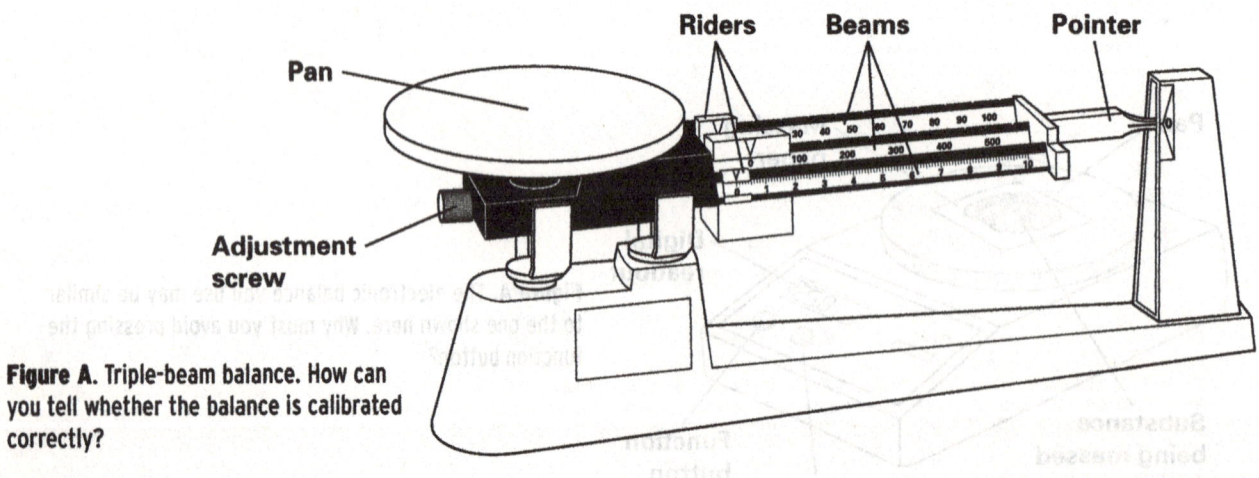

Figure A. Triple-beam balance. How can you tell whether the balance is calibrated correctly?

To mass a substance, use the following procedure:
1. Place the material to be massed in a container on the pan.
2. Move the rider along the beam marked with the highest values until the pointer indicates midpoint. Again, the pointer doesn't need to stop swinging, but the swing should be an equal distance above and below the midpoint. If the beams are notched, make sure each rider sits in a notch.
3. Repeat Step 2 with the other beams.
4. To take a reading, add the masses indicated by the riders. **Figures B** and **C** show how to take a reading.

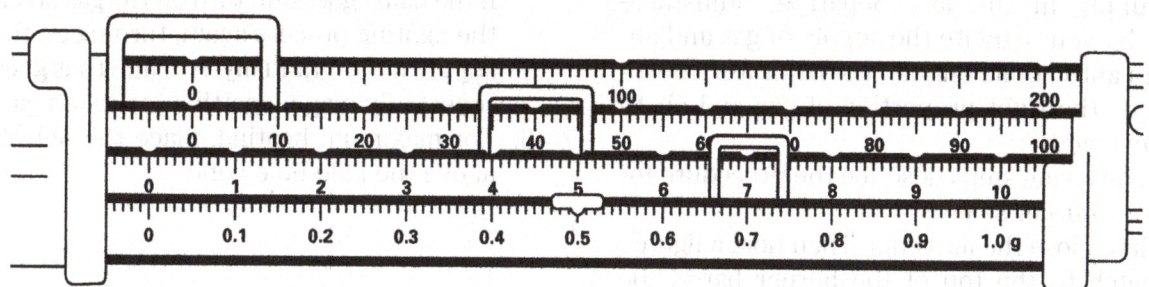

Figure B. This drawing shows four beams on a balance. The mass of the substance is the sum of the masses indicated on the beams. The mass shown here is 47.50 g.

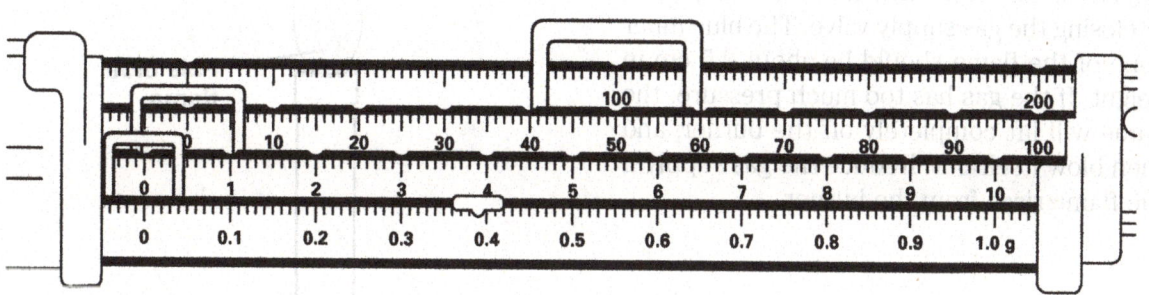

Figure C. Here you see four beams on a balance. What is the mass of the substance on this balance?

Food Science Lab Manual
Copyright © Mehas & Rodgers

Lighting a Laboratory Burner

A common item of equipment in the food science lab is the laboratory burner. Understanding how it works will enable you to use it efficiently and safely.

Most laboratory burners have the same basic parts (**Figure A**). A gas inlet connects with the gas supply in the lab. Separate, adjustable valves let you regulate the supply of gas and air. Like an automobile engine, the laboratory burner needs the right proportion of gas and air to work correctly.

The following steps describe the procedure for lighting a burner safely:

1. First, close the air vents. Then hold a lighted match to the top of the burner barrel. *Be sure you do this before turning on the gas supply.* Lighting the match when gas is already present may ignite an uncontrollable flame.
2. Slowly turn on the gas.
3. Adjust the size of the flame. Do this by opening or closing the gas supply valve. The blue inner cone of the flame should be about 2.5 cm in height. If the gas has too much pressure, the flame will lift completely off the burner, and then blow itself out. Reduce the gas supply if the flame rises from the burner.
4. Adjust the color of the flame. Do this by turning the burner barrel that controls the air supply. The inner flame should be pale blue. The outer and upper part of the flame should be pale violet. If the flame burns yellow, turn the barrel to increase the air supply.
5. If the flame goes out, turn off the gas and begin the lighting process again, turning on the gas supply more gradually. A flame that goes out repeatedly may be getting too much gas.
6. For maximum heating, place the object just above the pale blue cone.

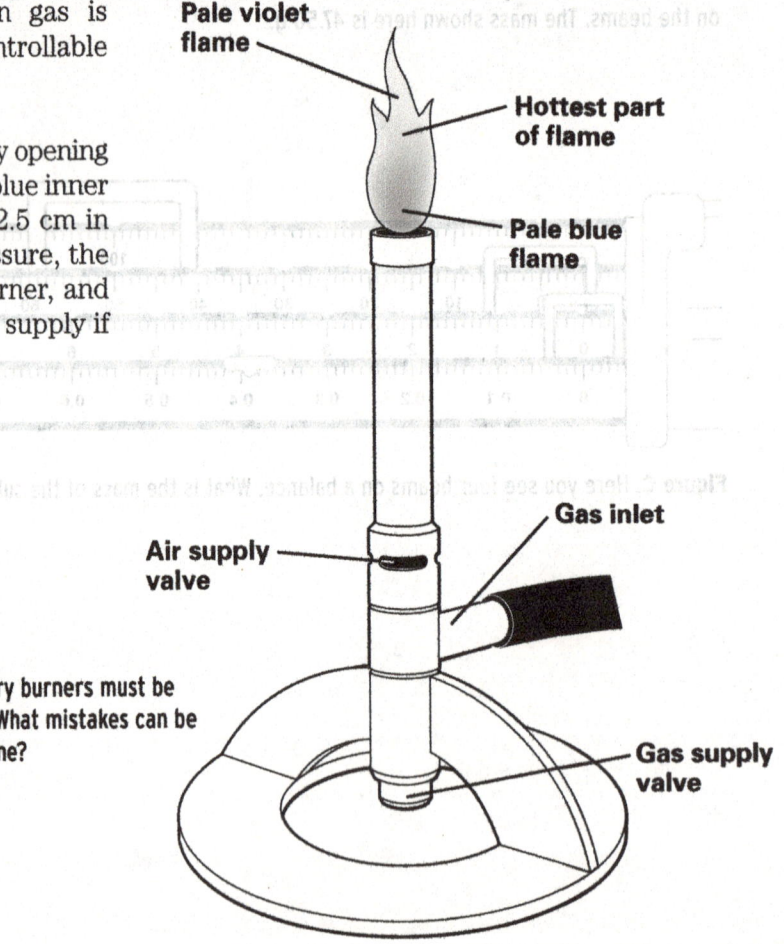

Figure A. Laboratory burners must be handled with care. What mistakes can be made when using one?

Using a Microscope

Some amazing things that happen in food science are beyond the scope of the human eye. A colony of tiny organisms can multiply to make bread rise—or to produce mold. Skill in using a microscope helps you appreciate and understand the activity of single-cell organisms in foods.

The pointers below can help you use a microscope appropriately. They will make more sense as you actually use the microscope and become familiar with the parts labeled in **Figure A**.

Tips for Microscope Use

- Store the microscope protected from dust, either in a cabinet or covered with cloth or plastic. Store with the low-power objective in place.
- Carry the microscope upright using both hands. One hand supports the base; the other holds the microscope arm.
- Always bring a specimen into focus with the low-power objective first.
- Never use the coarse adjustment to focus the high-power objective.
- When using the coarse adjustment to lower the low-power objective, always look at the microscope from the side. If you look through the eyepiece, you may accidentally force the objective into the coverslip, causing it to break. (The coverslip is a very thin piece of glass that is placed over the substance on the slide.)
- Avoid letting direct sunlight shine on the mirror; it may reflect up into the eye.
- Clean the lenses with lens paper only. If the lens does not wipe clean with dry paper, moisten with a drop of water or rubbing alcohol.
- Handle coverslips and microscope slides with care to avoid cracking and shattering.

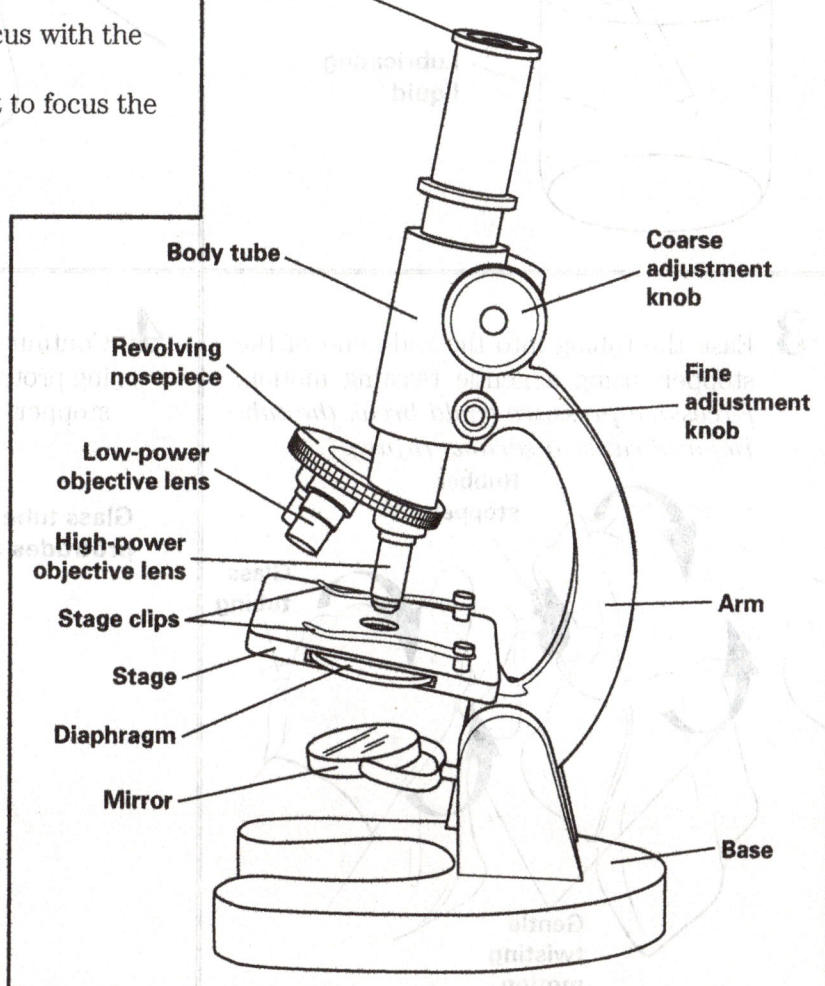

Figure A. Most microscopes have the parts listed here. What is the function of each part?

Food Science Lab Manual

Inserting Glass Tubing into a Rubber Stopper

You may recall that to measure the temperature of a liquid, a thermometer must be suspended in the middle of the fluid. This and similar techniques in food science call for inserting a thermometer or a length of glass tubing into a rubber stopper. A safe and successful procedure is outlined in the steps that follow.

1 Dip the tip of the glass tubing in a lubricating liquid, such as soapy water or glycerol.

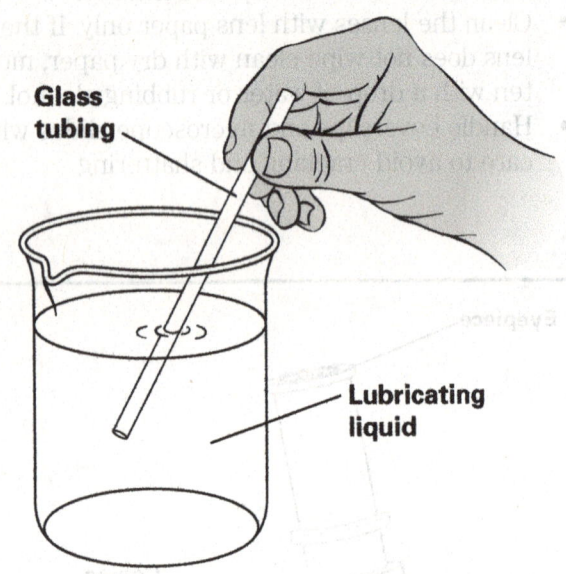

2 Protect your hands with cloth toweling as you encircle the stopper with your fingers. This hold prevents possible injury from pushing the end of the tubing into your palm.

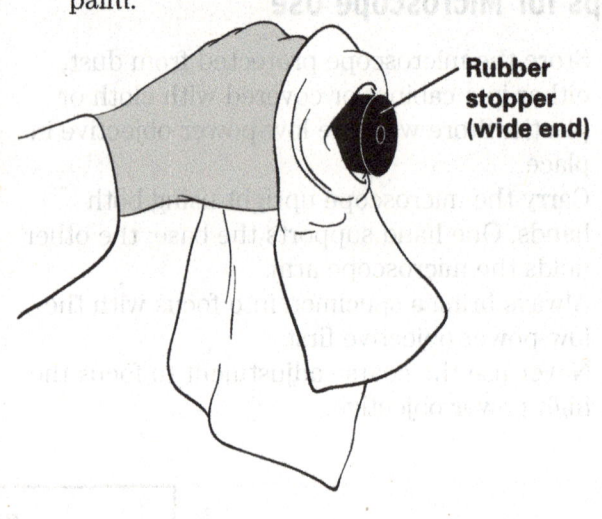

3 Ease the tubing into the wide end of the stopper, using a gentle twisting motion. *Excessive pressure could break the tubing and cause a serious injury.*

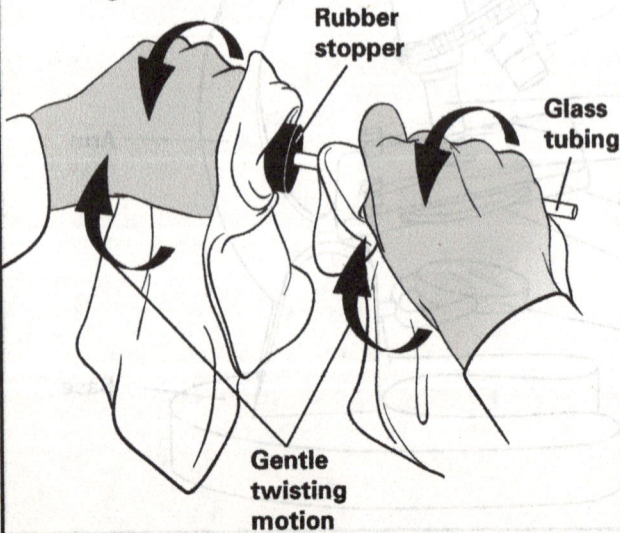

4 Continue twisting until the end of the tubing protrudes from the opposite end of the stopper.

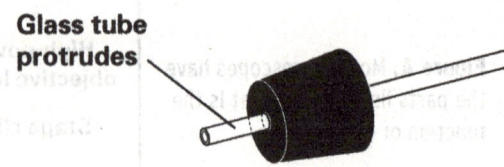

Using a Buret

Another useful piece of equipment in the food science lab is the buret. A buret is a specially designed, graduated tube. A buret is clamped to a ring stand and suspended over a container (**Figure A**). Liquid is added to the buret at the top. A valve, called a stopcock, lets you release the liquid from the buret drop by drop into another liquid in the container below.

You can fill a buret to any point on its scale, that is, anywhere from 0.00 to 50.00 mL. The 0 point is at the top of the scale so that you can easily determine how much liquid has been dispensed from the buret during an experiment.

Burets are used in titrations as well as other procedures. The following guidelines will help you use the buret for experiments in the food science lab:

- When setting up a buret, first make sure the stopcock works easily. If the mechanism sticks, report this to your teacher so the problem can be corrected.
- If you use a funnel to fill the buret, hold the funnel in your hand. Don't rest it on the buret.
- When adding solution to the buret, be sure to fill the tip. Open the stopcock slightly to let the liquid fill the tip from the main tube above.
- Once the buret is in place on the stand, place a beaker underneath to catch any excess liquid that is discharged when you fill the tip or lower the liquid from above zero to the zero line.
- When turning the stopcock, maintain a slight inward pressure. This will prevent solution from leaking around the stopcock plug.
- Be sure to read and record values on a buret accurately; you will need them to make calculations in an experiment.

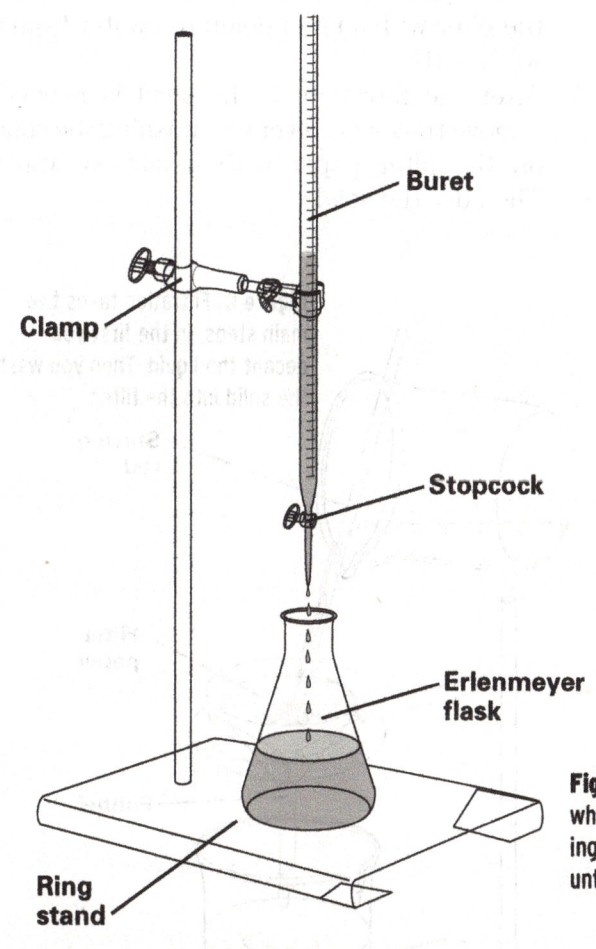

Figure A. With a buret, you can control the rate at which one solution is added to another. Practice filling a buret with water and adjusting the stopcock until you can release one drop at a time.

Filtering Substances

Some experiments in food science require separating the solid particles from a liquid. This is commonly done by filtration, which means pouring the liquid through a porous material (filter paper) that catches the solid particles. The process is described here.

1. Fold a circular piece of filter paper into a cone, as shown in the illustration (**Figure A**).
2. Set the cone in a filter funnel. Moisten the filter paper with a small amount of deionized water, pressing the paper gently to make it fit firmly against the funnel.
3. Place the funnel in an iron ring clamped to a ring stand. The tip of the funnel should touch the inside surface of the beaker and extend about 2.5 cm below the rim.
4. Place a beaker beneath the funnel to collect the filtrate, the liquid that passes through the funnel.
5. Next, decant the liquid. The principle of decanting is shown in **Figure B**. Decant the liquid from the solid by pouring the liquid down a glass stirring rod into the funnel. Be careful to keep the liquid below the top edge of the filter paper cone at all times; the liquid must not overflow (**Figure C**).

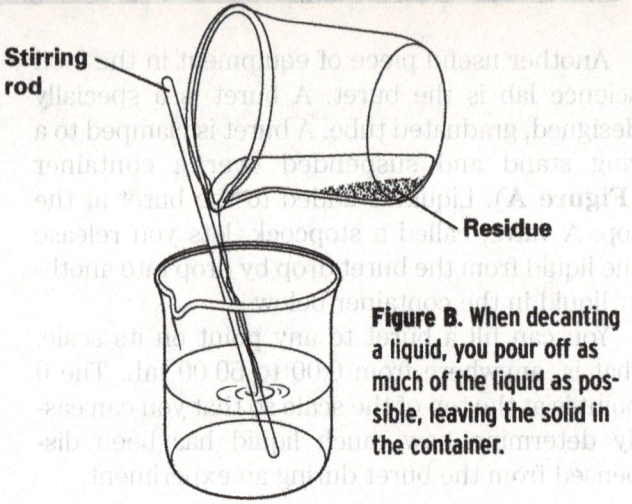

Figure B. When decanting a liquid, you pour off as much of the liquid as possible, leaving the solid in the container.

6. To complete the filtration, wash the solid into the filter with a jet of deionized water from a wash bottle.
7. After the filtration, if the solid is needed, remove traces of solvent by washing the solid on the filter paper with deionized water. Then dry the solid.

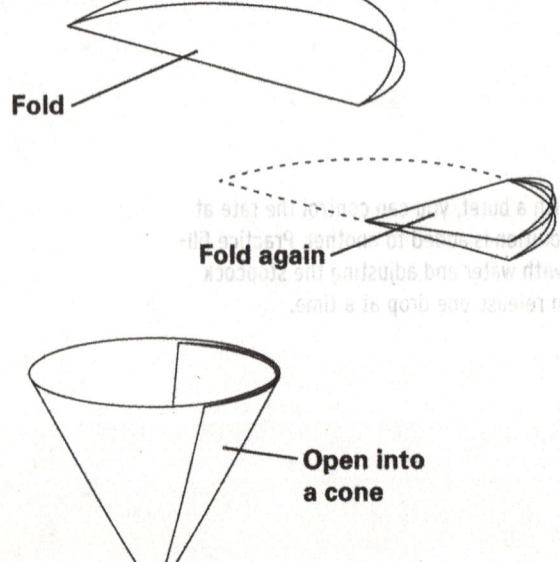

Figure A. To create a cone from the filter paper, fold the circle in half and then quarters. Open it into a cone by pulling three layers of paper to one side.

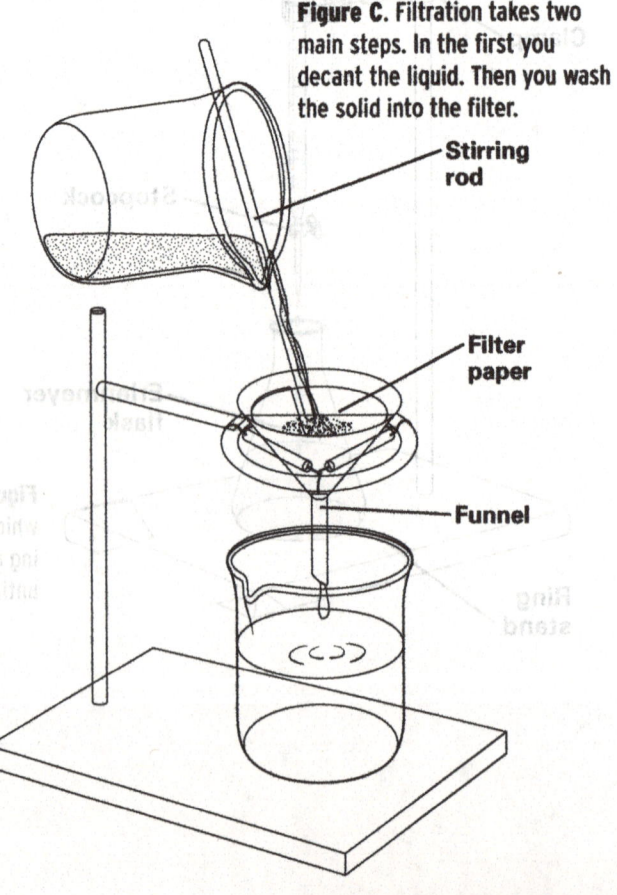

Figure C. Filtration takes two main steps. In the first you decant the liquid. Then you wash the solid into the filter.

Name _____ Date _____ Class _____

Using the Scientific Method

Directions: Do you know someone who likes to test ideas personally before accepting them? That investigative attitude is the basis for the scientific method of inquiry, described below. Read about the method and answer the questions that follow.

The Scientific Method

1. **Form a hypothesis.** State exactly what you want to demonstrate. What do you think will happen?
   - Gather information. A hypothesis is suggested by facts gained from research.
   - Use reasoning skills. A hypothesis follows logically from the facts.
2. **Test the hypothesis through experimentation.** Devise and carry out a test of your theory.
   - Control variables. Eliminate factors that could interfere with the purpose of the experiment.
3. **Analyze data.** Record and examine the results. Do they tend to support or disprove your hypothesis?
4. **Report your results.** Share findings with others in the scientific community.

The Scientific Method in Action

Scientists observed that white mice that were fed seeds appeared to grow more than mice given leafy green and yellow vegetables. The scientists hypothesized that the protein in the seed was responsible for the growth. They designed an experiment to test this hypothesis. They divided 200 mice of the same age, size, health, and gender into two groups of 100 mice each. The mice were kept under identical conditions for fourteen days. One group was given a diet low in protein. The other group was given a normal protein diet. The mass of each mouse was recorded daily for fourteen days.

(Continued on next page)

Food Science Lab Manual
Copyright © Mehas & Rodgers

About the Experiment

1. Which group of mice served as a control?
   _____
   _____

2. What was the variable?
   _____

3. What effect of the protein diet was tested?
   _____
   _____

4. What other effect of a protein diet could have been tested?
   _____
   _____

5. Why did scientists use a large number of mice in this experiment?
   _____
   _____

6. If the results of the experiment did not show a marked difference between the two groups, what should the scientists do next?
   _____
   _____
   _____
   _____

Name _____ Date _____ Class _____

Evaluating Laboratory Situations

Directions: Using guidelines from this manual and your own lab experience, evaluate the situations described below. Is the action a safe one? Will the procedure be successful? Would you do anything differently? Write and explain your response on the lines provided.

1. While Cal and his lab partner were conducting an experiment, Cal held the test tube rack toward Ramon. "Look in this test tube," Cal said. "The smoke is turning pink!"

   _____
   _____
   _____
   _____
   _____

2. During an experiment, Stephen began heating a solution in a beaker. To take the solution's temperature, he leaned the thermometer against the side of the beaker while he read the rest of the instructions.

   _____
   _____
   _____
   _____
   _____

3. Reiko took off her hoop earrings and put them in her purse when she entered the lab. She set her purse under the table in her work area.

   _____
   _____
   _____
   _____
   _____

(Continued on next page)

4. Kirk struck a match and held it next to a laboratory burner. Then he opened the burner gas valve.

_____
_____
_____

5. Marguerite needed to plug her electric mixer into an electrical outlet in order to complete a lab experiment, but the closest electrical outlet was already in use. She stretched the cord across the sink to reach another outlet.

_____
_____
_____
_____
_____

6. Derek misplaced the massing paper he had used to mass a substance at the start of an experiment. For a later step in the experiment, he massed a substance on a piece of notebook paper that appeared to be about the same size as the lost massing paper.

_____
_____
_____
_____
_____

7. Brittany burned her arm on a hotplate. She wrapped it with a damp paper towel until she finished her experiment.

_____
_____
_____
_____
_____

(Continued on next page)

Name _____ Date _____ Class _____

Evaluating Laboratory Situations (Continued)

8. When his experiment failed to support his hypothesis, Alex tried the procedure again. When he got the same results, he concluded his hypothesis was incorrect.

   _____
   _____
   _____
   _____
   _____

9. As a joke, Lisa put a small plastic spider in the food her lab partner was about to taste test.

   _____
   _____
   _____
   _____
   _____

Name _____ Date _____ Class _____

Estimating Metric Measurements

Science deals with exact values, but learning to estimate those values is a useful skill. Having a rough idea of what result to expect can guide your calculations and alert you to errors along the way. For science, you need to translate English measurements—feet, cups, and pounds—into metric units—centimeters, liters, grams, and more.

Part I

Directions: For each item below, estimate the value requested, using a suitable metric unit. Then answer the questions that follow.

	Estimated Value	Actual Value
1. How long, tall, or far is … ?		
a. a paper clip		
b. your classroom door		
c. your arm and hand		
d. the floor from the ceiling		
2. What is the mass of … ?		
a. one chocolate chip		
b. one saltine cracker		
c. your food science text		
d. your shoe		
3. What is the volume held by … ?		
a. a soup spoon		
b. a school lunch milk carton		
c. a coffee mug		
d. a soft drink can		

(Continued on next page)

Food Science Lab Manual
Copyright © Mehas & Rodgers

	Estimated Value	Actual Value

4. What is the temperature of … ?

    a. a cup of cold tap water

    b. a cup of hot tap water

    c. refrigerated soft drinks

    d. a cup of hot cocoa

5. For which type of measurement were your estimates most accurate? Least accurate?

_____

_____

6. Why might some measurements be easier to estimate than others?

_____

_____

_____

_____

Part II

Directions: Repeat the directions in Part I for the items below. Then compare the results to those from Part I to answer the questions that follow.

	Estimated Value	Actual Value

1. How long, tall, or far is … ?

    a. a dollar bill

    b. your sleeve

    c. the height of the bulletin board

    d. this room from the nearest exit

2. What is the mass of … ?

    a. one potato chip

    b. one student's purse

    c. a pencil

    d. a 2-L bottle of soft drink

(Continued on next page)

Name _____ Date _____ Class _____

Estimating Metric Measurements (Continued)

	Estimated Value	Actual Value
3. What is the volume held by ... ?		
a. a drinking straw	_____	_____
b. a "juice box"	_____	_____
c. a cereal bowl	_____	_____
d. a 6-cm depth in the lab sink	_____	_____
4. What is the temperature of ... ?		
a. a glass of ice water	_____	_____
b. a cup of coffee	_____	_____
c. water sitting outdoors	_____	_____
d. heated, bubbling water	_____	_____

5. For which types of values did your estimating skills most improve?

   _____

   _____

6. List three practical benefits of developing estimating skills.

   _____

   _____

   _____

   _____

7. List two common activities you can use to practice your estimating skills.

   _____

   _____

   _____

   _____

Food Science Lab Manual
Copyright © Mehas & Rodgers

Name _____ Date _____ Class _____

Creating Line Graphs

Directions: A line graph is one type of graph that presents data as plotted points connected by a line. These graphs are useful for illustrating slow changes, as shown in the world population example below. Study the line graph example below on world population. Then use the information provided to create a line graph of your own.

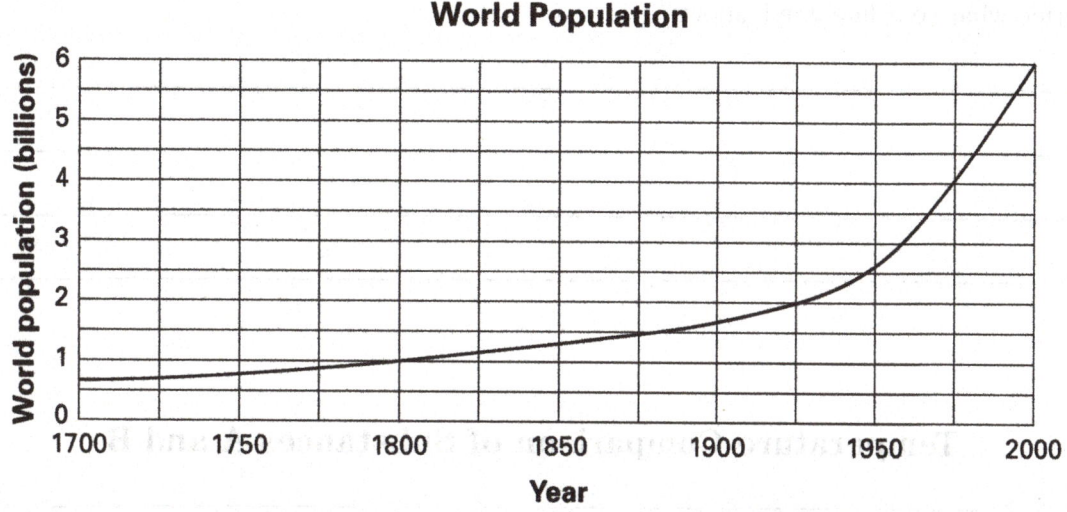

Recording Temperatures with a Line Graph

Suppose you measure the temperature of two substances during an experiment. *Both substances, A and B, begin with a temperature of 20°C.* The remaining readings are as follows:

- **Substance A.** After one minute, you record a temperature of 28°C. At one-minute intervals thereafter, you record 40, 47, 55, 62, 88, 91, 98, and 100°C.

- **Substance B.** After one minute, you record a temperature of 32°C. At one-minute intervals thereafter, you record 43, 48, 51, 60, 68, 75, 79, and 84°C.

Using the blank grid provided, plot a line graph that shows how the temperatures of the two different substances changed at one-minute intervals during the experiment. Plot time horizontally, with two blocks representing a minute. Plot temperature vertically, with one block representing 10°C. Connect the points with straight lines, using dotted lines for substance B.

(Continued on next page)

Food Science Lab Manual
Copyright © Mehas & Rodgers

Analyzing Your Graph

1. Both substances began with the same temperature. Did they ever have the same temperature again? Explain.

   _____

   _____

   _____

2. Describe what your line graph shows.

   _____

   _____

   _____

   _____

   _____

Temperature Comparison of Substances A and B

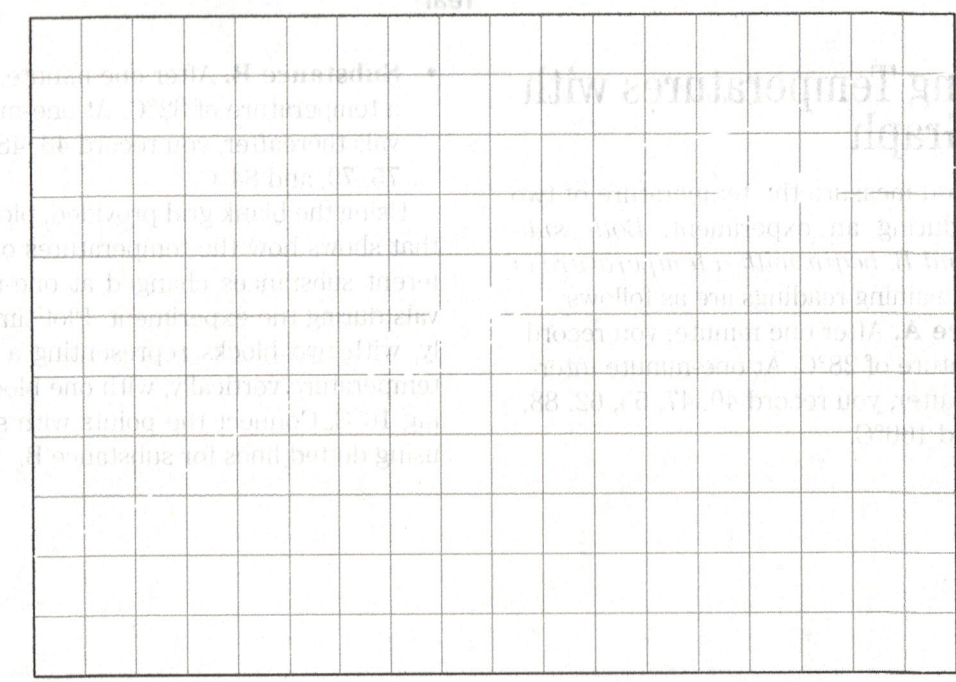

Name _____ Date _____ Class _____

Creating Tables

Directions: Every time you read a grade report, a bus schedule, or the score of a ball game, you use a table. Tables present information clearly, making them an efficient way to communicate data. In this course, you'll be asked to read and create tables. After reading about tables below, use the information provided to create one of your own.

Parts of a Table

Tables like the example shown here have four main parts.
- The *title* runs across the top and tells what information the table contains.
- *Columns* are the sections that run down the table.
- A *column head* identifies the information found in that column. Often the first column on the left lists items that the other columns describe.
- *Rows* are read from left to right.

Nutritional Information on Selected Cheeses

Food (28.35 g, or 1 ounce)	Kcalories	Total Fat (g)	Saturated Fat (g)	Protein (g)	Calcium (mg)
American cheese	105	9	5.5	6	172
Blue cheese	99	8	5.2	6	148
Cheddar cheese	113	9	5.9	7	202
Mozzarella (whole milk)	79	6	3.7	5	145
Parmesan	128	8	5.5	12	385
Swiss cheese	105	8	5	8	269

(Continued on next page)

Food Science Lab Manual
Copyright © Mehas & Rodgers

To construct a table, you need to decide what information you want to include and how best to communicate it. Those decisions will help you choose a title, write column heads, and develop a format that includes the correct number of rows and columns.

Constructing a Table on Lab Supplies

Suppose your class will be conducting two experiments. You need the following quantities of different chemical substances (identified as A-E):
Experiment 1: A—0.50 g; B—0.0 g; C—2.10 g; D—8.70 mL; and E—6.0 mL.
Experiment 2: A—1.25 g; B—3.60 g; C—0.0 g; D—45.7 mL; and E—12.5 mL.

Your lab has the following amounts of each substance already on hand: A—30.0 g; B—30.0 g; C—23.0 g; D—138 mL; and E—1 L.

Twelve groups in your class will each perform both experiments. Calculate how much of each substance the twelve groups will need in total for both experiments. Also calculate how much more of each substance the class needs in addition to what is already available in the lab. Arrange all information in the blank table below. You may want to organize your plan on scrap paper first.

Substance	Amount Needed for Experiment 1	Amount Needed for Experiment 2	Total Amount Needed for 12 Student Groups	Amount on Hand	Additional Amount Needed

46

Food Science Lab Manual
Copyright © Mehas & Rodgers

Creating Bar Graphs

Directions. A bar graph conveys information with solid bars. Suppose you want to compare experiment results to those of another lab group. A graph with different colored bars might do the job. Note the fat comparisons made in the sample bar graph below. Then work with others to create the bar graphs described.

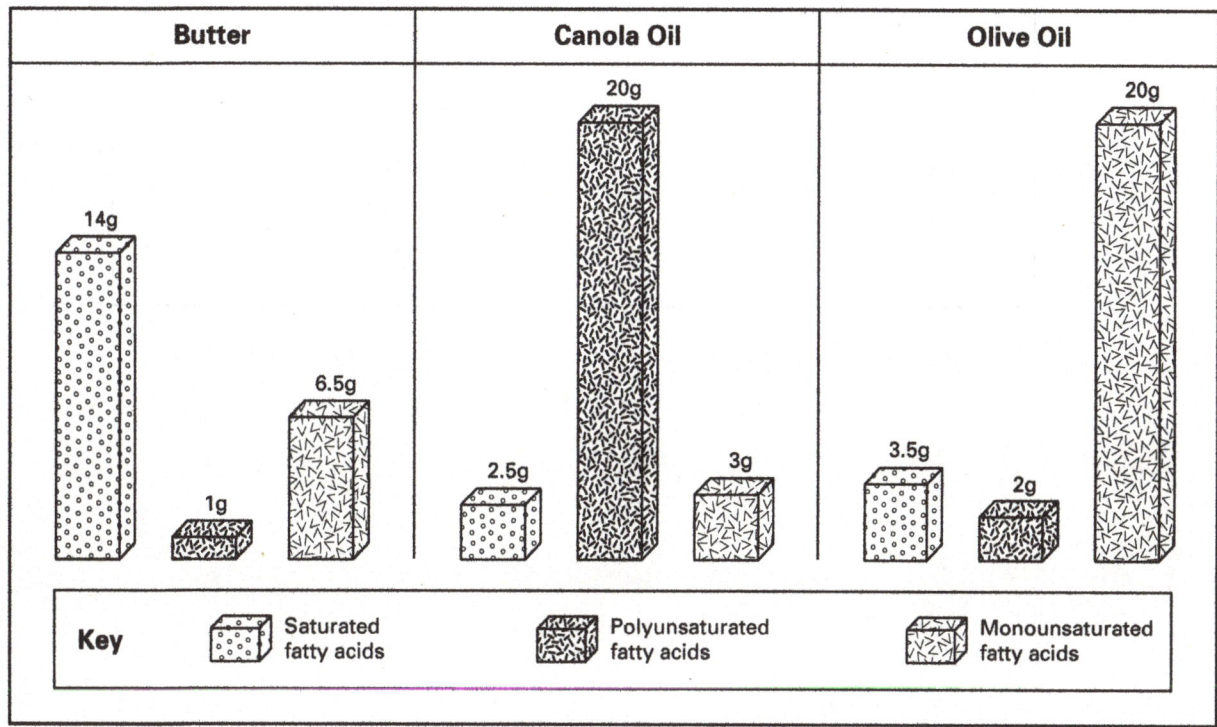

Creating a Bar Graph Showing Folate in Foods

Work with a group of several students to create bar graphs that show the folate content in selected foods. Divide responsibility for making a separate graph for each of the different groups in the Food Guide Pyramid, making fruits and vegetables into two separate graphs. In each graph show the folate content of 6-10 selected foods from that group. For example, the person(s) graphing the vegetable group might include the folate content in micrograms for carrots, spinach, broccoli, asparagus, etc.

When done, compare graphs. Then work together to create one bar graph that compares folate content in the different food groups.

Note that male teens need 300 micrograms of folate daily. Female teens and all adults need 400. Pregnant females need 600.

(Continued on next page)

Food Science Lab Manual
Copyright © Mehas & Rodgers

Creating Bar Graphs

Directions. A bar graph conveys information with solid bars. Suppose you want to compare experiment results to those of another lab group. A graph with different colored bars might do the job. Note the fat comparisons made in the sample bar graph below. Then work with others to create the bar graphs described.

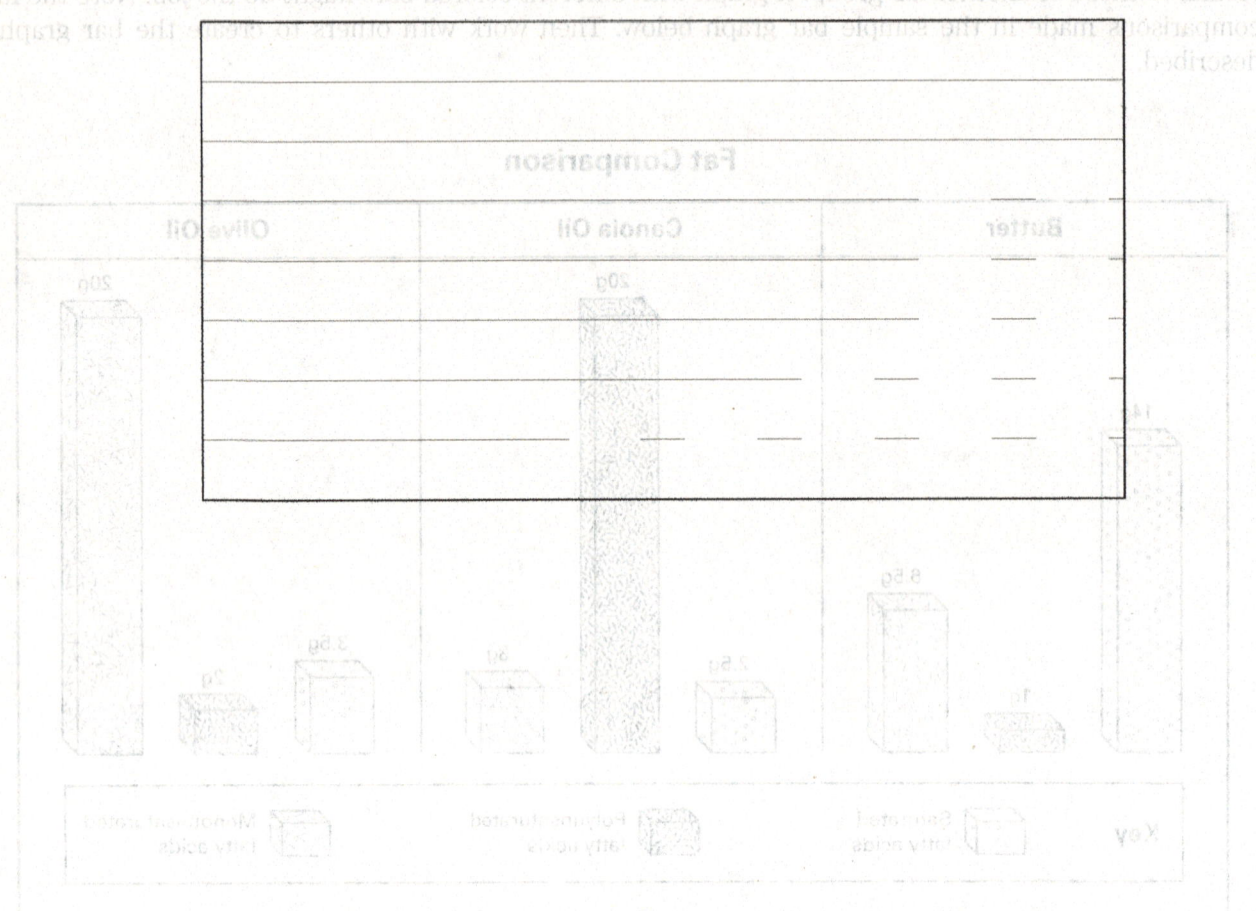

Creating a Bar Graph Showing Folate in Foods

Work with a group of several students to create bar graphs that show the folate content in selected foods. Divide responsibility for making a separate graph for each of the different groups in the Food Guide Pyramid, making fruits and vegetables into two separate graphs. In each graph show the folate content of 5-10 selected foods from that group. For example, the person(s) graphing the vegetable group might include the folate content in milligrams for carrots, spinach, broccoli, asparagus, etc.

When done, compare graphs. Then work together to create one bar graph that compares folate content in the different food groups.

Note that male teens need 200 micrograms of folate daily. Female teens and all adults need 400. Pregnant females need 800

(Continued on next page)

48 Food Science Lab Manual
Copyright © Mehas & Rodgers

Name _____ Date _____ Class _____

Creating Pie Charts

Directions: A pie chart is convenient for showing percentages visually. Values appear as wedges of a pie, cut in proportion and totaling 100 percent. Sections are individually labeled and often differently colored. Examine the pie chart shown here and then create one of your own, using the information below.

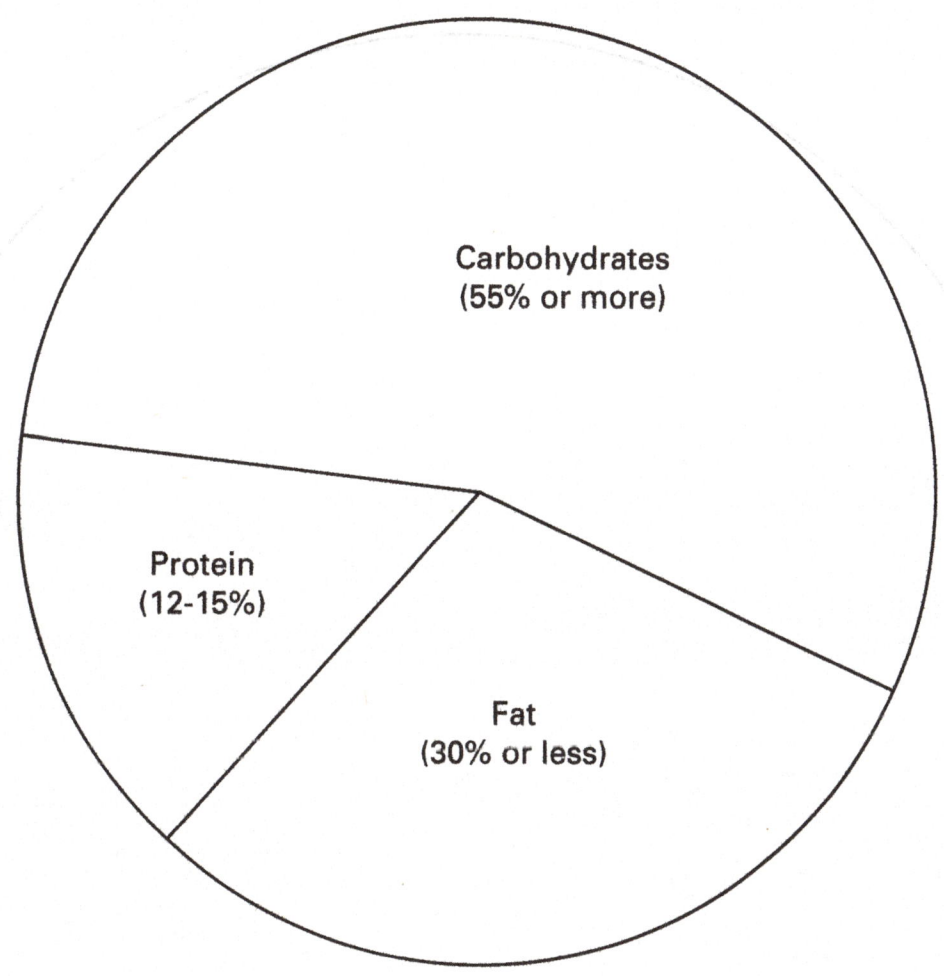

Recommended Calorie Sources
- Carbohydrates (55% or more)
- Protein (12-15%)
- Fat (30% or less)

Creating a Pie Chart with a Protractor

When making a pie chart, you may be able to estimate how large to make each wedge. To determine the exact size, however, you can use a formula. Divide the number that one wedge will represent by the number shown by the whole pie. Then multiply the result by 360, the number of degrees in a circle. This tells the angle to draw for that wedge.

(Continued on next page)

Food Science Lab Manual
Copyright © Mehas & Rodgers

Using a protractor and the formula just described, create a pie chart from the blank one provided here. The chart should show the following average number of servings that nutritionists recommend in a teen's daily diet: nine servings of grain and cereal products; four servings of vegetables; four servings of fruit; three servings of dairy products; and two servings of meat or poultry. Remember to title your graph. The value for grain and cereal products has been figured as a model.

Total number of servings = 22
Number of grain and cereal product servings = 9
9 ÷ 22 = 0.4090 × 360 = 147.2
Grain and cereal products servings = 147° angle

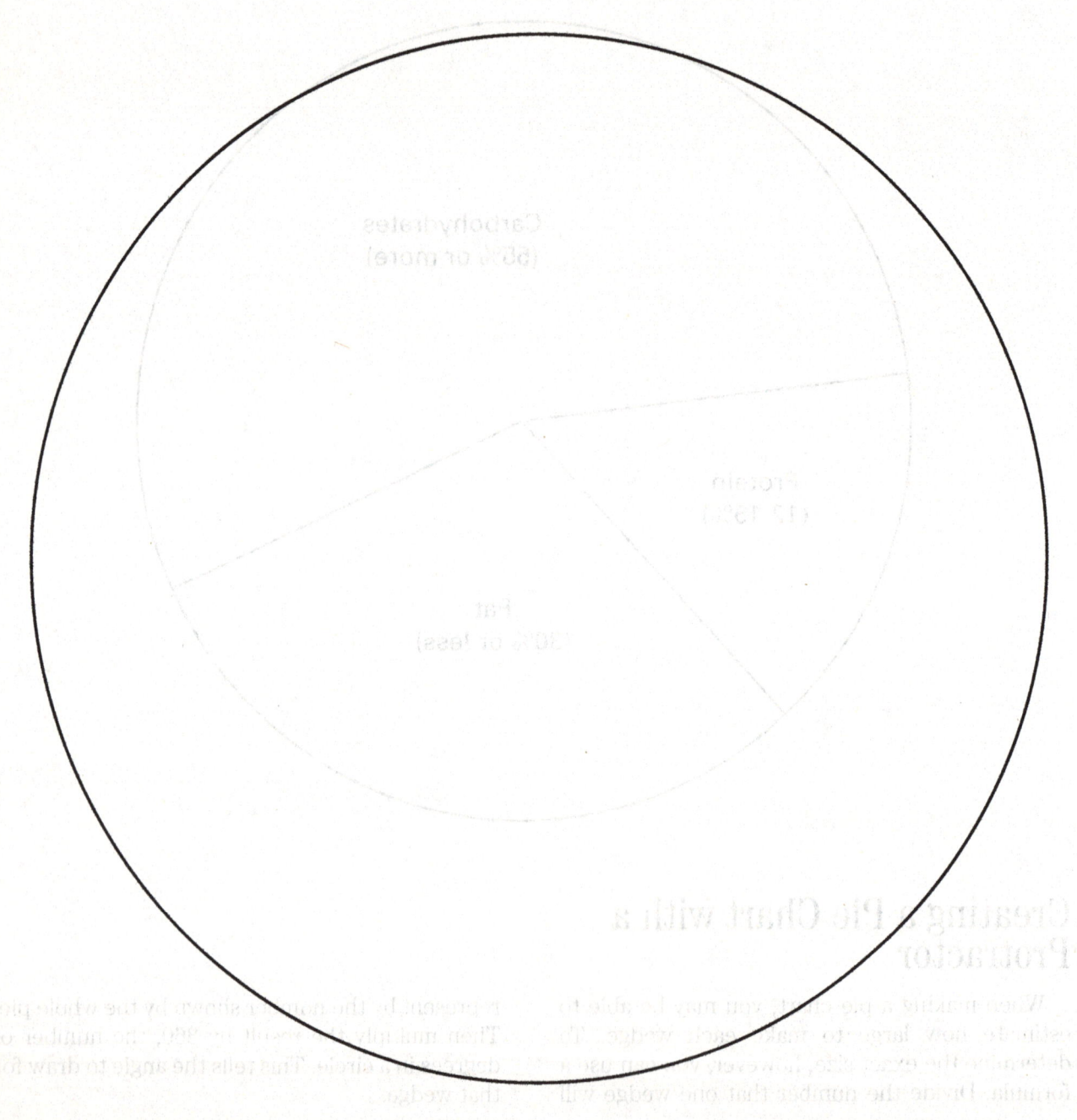

Name _____ Date _____ Class _____

Food Labels and Nutrition

EXPERIMENT 2-1

Nearly all packaged foods sold in the United States are required by law to display nutritional information on their containers for the benefit of consumers. You can find this information on the Nutrition Facts panel typically printed on the side or back of a package. Food scientists have contributed to the formulation of this information.

Although you'll learn more in Unit 4 about the meaning of terms on a Nutrition Facts panel, you can start to become familiar with the data now. To begin evaluating the contributions of food science to your diet, compare the labels on two products that appear regularly at many breakfast tables.

Equipment and Materials
Nutrition Facts panels from two different food packages

Procedure
1. Obtain one Nutrition Facts panel from a container of oatmeal and one from a container of ready-to-eat cereal from your teacher. (Use other products for comparison if your teacher provides different ones.)
2. In your data table, identify the products you're using.
3. Examine the Nutrition Facts panel on each product and record the information called for in your data table.

Analyzing Results

1. How do the foods compare in calories, total fat, and cholesterol?

_____
_____
_____
_____

2. Which food was higher in sodium and sugar?

_____
_____

3. Which of the two products was higher in vitamins and minerals?

_____
_____

(Continued on next page)

Food Science Lab Manual
Copyright © Mehas & Rodgers

EXPERIMENT 2-1 (Continued)

4. How do you account for differences in nutritional value?

5. Based on your current understanding of nutrition, what advantages and disadvantages do you see in eating each food item?

DATA TABLE

	Product One		Product Two	
Nutrient	**Amount per Serving**	**% Daily Value**	**Amount per Serving**	**% Daily Value**
Calories				
Total fat				
Cholesterol				
Sodium				
Dietary fiber				
Sugars				
Protein				
Vitamins (List)				
Minerals (List)				

Food Science Lab Manual
Copyright © Mehas & Rodgers

Name _____ Date _____ Class _____

Packaged Food Scavenger Hunt

EXPERIMENT 2-2

SAFETY FIRST
Review these safety guidelines before you begin this experiment.

In this activity you will explore the shelves of a grocery store, looking for food items that fit the descriptions given.

Equipment and Materials
paper   pen or pencil

Procedure

Food	Preservation Techniques		
a.			
b.			
c.			

1. Find three foods, each of which has been preserved using three different techniques, including drying, freezing, canning, freeze-drying, and fermentation. Write these in the chart above.

2. Identify by type and brand name a freeze-dried food other than coffee.

   a. Food Item: _____

   b. Brand: _____

3. List six food items that contain imitation flavors.

   a. _____

   b. _____

   c. _____

   d. _____

   e. _____

   f. _____

(Continued on next page)

Food Science Lab Manual
Copyright © Mehas & Rodgers

EXPERIMENT 2-2 (Continued)

4. List six food items that contain artificial colors.

   a. _____

   b. _____

   c. _____

   d. _____

   e. _____

   f. _____

5. Find three imitation meat items.

   a. _____

   b. _____

   c. _____

6. Locate two items stored in aseptic packaging.

   a. _____

   b. _____

Analyzing Results

1. Were any items hard to find? If so, which ones?

   _____

   _____

   _____

2. What type of food processing seems most commonly used?

   _____

3. How does the amount of processed foods compare with the amount of fresh foods available? Why do you think this situation exists?

   _____

   _____

   _____

   _____

4. From this survey, what can you conclude about the role of processing in the food supply?

   _____

   _____

   _____

   _____

Food Science Lab Manual
Copyright © Mehas & Rodgers

Name _____ Date _____ Class _____

Using an Electronic Balance

EXPERIMENT 3-1

SAFETY FIRST
Review these safety guidelines before you begin this experiment.

One of the first skills you need to learn in food science is how to use a balance, the instrument used to mass materials. One type of balance often used in science laboratories is the electronic balance. An electronic balance has a pan similar to those found on a triple-beam balance, but no arms or beams.

On the front of most electronic balances are two buttons called sensors. One is labeled "function" and the other is labeled "tare." Don't press the function button unless instructed to do so by your teacher, since it will change the units in which the mass of your sample will be reported. The tare button will be very useful when you mass a sample on paper or in a container. Pressing the button sets the balance to zero. You will learn to use the tare button in conducting this experiment.

Equipment and Materials

3 items to mass
electronic balance
massing paper
5-mL measuring spoon
straightedge spatula
table salt

Procedure

1. From your teacher, obtain three items to mass.
2. Place one of the items on the balance pan or platform. Read the mass of the item on the screen at the front of the balance.
3. In your data table, record the name of the item and its mass.
4. Mass each of the other items and record the information in your data table.
5. Place a piece of massing or waxed paper on the balance pan or platform. Press the tare button. The balance will cancel the mass of the paper so that the screen reads zero.
6. Fill a 5-mL measuring spoon with table salt. Level it with a straightedge spatula.
7. Pour the salt onto the paper. Read the mass of the salt on the screen.
8. Record the mass of the salt in your data table.

Analyzing Results

1. How does the mass of each item you used compare to its size?

_____
_____
_____
_____
_____

(Continued on next page)

Food Science Lab Manual
Copyright © Mehas & Rodgers

EXPERIMENT 3-1 (Continued)

2. In what aspects of food production do you think taring is used?

_____

_____

_____

DATA TABLE

Item	Mass
5 mL table salt	

_____

_____

_____

_____

_____

_____

56   **Food Science Lab Manual**
Copyright © Mehas & Rodgers

Name _____ Date _____ Class _____

Precision in Measurement

EXPERIMENT 3-2

SAFETY FIRST
Review these safety guidelines before you begin this experiment.

In all areas of science, measuring quantities of materials precisely is of utmost importance. In this experiment, you will compare the masses of designated volumes of solids to determine whether measuring by mass or by volume gives more precise results.

Equipment and Materials

250-mL measuring cup
125-mL measuring cup
50-mL measuring cup

flour (variations 1 and 2)
brown sugar (variations 3 and 4)
balance

spoon
metal spatula
sifter

Procedure

1. Mass 250-mL, 125-mL, and 50-mL measuring cups individually. Record the masses in your data table.
2. Follow the variation assigned by your teacher.
   Variation 1. Lightly spoon all-purpose flour into the 250-mL measuring cup. Level the flour with the straight edge of a metal spatula. Mass the flour and cup. Using the same flour, repeat the procedure with the 125-mL cup, and then with the 50-mL cup. Record these values in your data table.
   Variation 2. Sift all-purpose flour. Lightly spoon the sifted flour into the 250-mL measuring cup. Level the flour with the straight edge of a metal spatula. Mass the flour and cup. Resift the flour. Repeat the procedure with the 125-mL cup, and then with the 50-mL cup. Record these values in your data table.
   Variation 3. Lightly spoon brown sugar into the 250-mL measuring cup. Level the cup with the straight edge of a metal spatula. Mass the brown sugar and cup. Using the same sugar, repeat the procedure with the 125-mL cup, and then with the 50-mL cup. Record these values in your data table.
   Variation 4. Firmly press brown sugar into the 250-mL measuring cup. Level the cup with the straight edge of a metal spatula. Mass the brown sugar and cup. Using the same sugar, repeat the procedure with the 125-mL cup, and then with the 50-mL cup. Record these values in your data table.
3. Determine the mass of each volume measured by subtracting the mass of the empty measuring cup from the mass of the cup and solid. Record the masses in your data table and on the board.
4. Average the results written on the board for each solid. Record these averaged values in your data table.

(Continued on next page)

EXPERIMENT 3-2 (Continued)

Analyzing Results

1. Multiply the average mass of each 50-mL measurement by 5 and each 125-mL measurement by 2. Which substance is closest in value to the mass of 250 mL as measured on the balance?

   _____

2. Which gave more precise results, the sifted or unsifted flour? The firmly pressed or lightly spooned brown sugar?

   _____

   _____

   _____

3. How do you explain the different degrees of precision among the different variations?

   _____

   _____

   _____

DATA TABLE

Variation Followed _____

Volume	Mass						
	Empty Cup	Cup and Solid	Solid	Average of Variations			
				#1	#2	#3	#4
250 mL							
125 mL							
50 mL							

58 Food Science Lab Manual
Copyright © Mehas & Rodgers

Measuring the Volume of a Liquid

EXPERIMENT 4-1

SAFETY FIRST
Review these safety guidelines before you begin this experiment.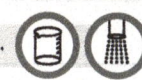

Using the proper equipment for experiments in the food science lab makes tasks easier and results more accurate. Liquid volumes can be measured with a beaker, graduated cylinder, or buret. In this experiment you'll compare the degree of accuracy allowed by these pieces of equipment.

Equipment and Materials
water	100-mL graduated cylinder	50-mL buret	utility clamp
150-mL beaker	10-mL graduated cylinder	ring stand	

Procedure

1. Go to the station assigned to you by your teacher. Read as precisely as you can the volume of liquid in the beaker, graduated cylinder, and the two burets at the station. Record your readings in your data table. Remember to read volumes from the bottom of the meniscus if you can see one.
2. Return to your own lab station. Using the gradations on the side of a 150-mL beaker, add exactly 45 mL of tap water to the beaker. Without spilling any, pour this water into a 100-mL graduated cylinder and read the volume to the nearest 0.1 mL. Record in your data table. Empty the graduated cylinder.
3. Using the gradations on the side of the beaker, add exactly 7 mL of tap water to the beaker. Without spilling any, pour this water into a 10-mL graduated cylinder and read the volume to the nearest 0.01 mL. Record in your data table. Empty the graduated cylinder.
4. Clamp a clean 50-mL buret to a ring stand, using a utility clamp. Fill the buret with tap water. It is best to add water above the zero line and then release water slowly into the beaker until the liquid in the buret is at or below the zero line. Discard the extra water.
5. Release exactly 22.00 mL of water from the buret into the 100-mL graduated cylinder. Read the volume of liquid in the graduated cylinder as precisely as you can and record in your data table.
6. Release 6.55 mL of water from the same buret into the 10-mL graduated cylinder. Read and record this amount as accurately as possible in your data table.

Analyzing Results

1. Based on the reading from the graduated cylinder, is a beaker suitable for measuring 45 mL of water? For measuring 7 mL of water?

_____

_____

_____

(Continued on next page)

EXPERIMENT 4-1 (Continued)

2. When, if ever, would you use a beaker to measure volumes of liquid in an experiment?
   _____
   _____
   _____

3. Compare your readings for the water released into each graduated cylinder. Which cylinder measured more accurately?
   _____
   _____
   _____

4. Do you think these same general results apply to measuring volumes of other types of substances, such as sand or oil? Why or why not?
   _____
   _____

DATA TABLE

Equipment	Volume	Station Number
Beaker		
Graduated cylinder		
Buret #1		
Buret #2		

VOLUME READINGS

Amount of Water	100-mL Graduated Cylinder	10-mL Graduated Cylinder
45 mL		
7 mL		
22 mL		
6.55 mL		

Name _____ Date _____ Class _____

Using a Graduated Cylinder

EXPERIMENT 4-2

SAFETY FIRST
Review these safety guidelines before you begin this experiment.

Volume is the amount of space material occupies. It can be determined in a number of ways. For objects such as a cube or a rectangular solid, you measure the length, width, and height, then multiply these values. In the food science lab, finding the volume of liquids is easier still. You simply pour the liquid into a container that is marked with volume measurements and read the level of the liquid.

In the lab, a graduated cylinder is often used to measure volume. Recall that it's important to read the volume from the meniscus, the bottom of the curve the liquid forms, and to estimate the volume to one-tenth of the smallest division of the scale marked on the cylinder.

Equipment and Materials
100-mL beaker   100-mL graduated cylinder   water

Procedure
1. Fill a 100-mL beaker with water to the 20-mL line.
2. Pour this water into a 100-mL graduated cylinder. Read and record the volume of the water in your data table.
3. Repeat Steps 1 and 2 with 30 mL of water.
4. Repeat Steps 1 and 2 with 25 mL of water. You will need to estimate this amount in the beaker.

Analyzing Results

1. How do the two readings of each volume compare between the beaker and the cylinder?

   _____
   _____
   _____

2. How do you explain any differences in each pair of readings?

   _____
   _____
   _____

(Continued on next page)

EXPERIMENT 4-2 (Continued)

3. Graduated cylinders cost three times as much as beakers of similar volumes. Why do you think this is so?

_____

_____

_____

DATA TABLE

Water	Beaker Reading	Graduated Cylinder Reading
20 mL		
30 mL		
25 mL		

(Continued on next page)

Mass and Volume of Beans

EXPERIMENT 4-3

SAFETY FIRST
Review these safety guidelines before you begin this experiment.

You are probably aware that many substances increase in volume by absorbing water. In this experiment, you will examine the volume and mass changes of various types of dried beans allowed to soak overnight in water. You will learn to measure the volume of irregular objects, such as beans, by determining how much water they take the place of. This is called measuring by water displacement.

Equipment and Materials
- 50 dried beans
- small beaker to hold 50 beans
- balance
- water
- 100-mL graduated cylinder
- brush for cleaning cylinder
- 100-mL beaker
- masking tape
- marking pen

Procedure

1. Count out 50 dried beans of the variety assigned by your teacher.
2. Mass a small beaker. Record this value in your data table.
3. Place the beans in the beaker and mass them. Record this value in your data table.
4. Determine the mass of the beans by subtracting the beaker's mass from the mass of the beaker and beans. Record this value in your data table.
5. Pour about 40 mL of water into a 100-mL graduated cylinder. Record the exact volume of water in your data table.
6. Carefully add the beans to the cylinder. Do not splash any of the water out of the cylinder.
7. Read the volume of the combined beans and water and record this in your data table.
8. Determine the volume of the 50 beans by subtracting the volume of water from the volume of combined beans and water. Record this value in your data table.
9. Transfer the beans to a 100-mL beaker, making sure no beans are left in the cylinder. Add enough water to fill the beaker. Label the beaker with your name and class. Store the beaker overnight on the tray specified by your teacher.
10. The following day, drain the beans thoroughly. Repeat Steps 2-8 with the soaked beans.
11. Calculate the mass of one dried bean and one soaked bean by dividing the total mass, found in Steps 4 and 8, by 50. Record these values in your data table.
12. Calculate and record the volume of one dried bean and one soaked bean.
13. Calculate the change in mass and the change in volume for one bean. Record in your data table.

(Continued on next page)

Food Science Lab Manual
Copyright © Mehas & Rodgers

EXPERIMENT 4-3 (Continued)

Analyzing Results

1. Compare the changes in mass and volume of one bean among the different varieties of beans used by other lab groups. Which variety gained the most mass and volume? The least?

   _____
   _____
   _____
   _____
   _____

2. Based on class experimental results, what recommendations can you make about soaking or cooking beans for a recipe?

   _____
   _____
   _____
   _____
   _____

3. In what other situations in food preparation might measuring by water displacement be useful?

   _____
   _____
   _____
   _____
   _____

(Continued on next page)

EXPERIMENT 4-3 (Continued)

DATA TABLE

Data for Dried Beans				
Mass			Volume	
Beaker alone		Water in cylinder	
Beaker and 50 beans		Water and 50 beans	
50 beans alone		50 beans alone	
One bean		One bean	
Data for Soaked Beans				
Mass			Volume	
Beaker alone		Volume of water in cylinder	
Beaker and 50 beans		Water and 50 beans	
50 beans alone		50 beans alone	
One bean		One bean	
Change in mass of one bean		Change in volume of one bean	

Food Science Lab Manual
Copyright © Mehas & Rodgers

Properties of Popping Corn

EXPERIMENT 5-1

SAFETY FIRST
Review these safety guidelines before you begin this experiment.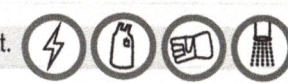

If you've ever popped popcorn, you know that some unpopped kernels often remain in the bottom of the popper. In this experiment, you'll try to determine what influences whether corn pops.

A little background will help you get started. Popcorn is bred for its water content; about 14 percent is considered ideal. As popcorn heats, the water inside each kernel expands. Pressure builds, causing the corn to pop. Knowing this, what is your hypothesis for this experiment?

Read through the experiment closely. Notice how the procedure is designed to control the variables.

Equipment and Materials

pin with plastic head
100 popcorn kernels for assigned variation
hot-air popcorn popper
bowl

Procedure

1. On the day before the experiment, help prepare kernels from a newly opened container of popcorn. Puncture some of the kernels of corn with a pin. Your teacher will place other kernels in a food dehydrator overnight to evaporate some of the water. The remainder of the sample will not be altered. This last group is called the control.
2. Follow the variation assigned by your teacher.
   Variation 1. Count out 100 kernels of unaltered popcorn.
   Variation 2. Count out 100 kernels of popcorn that has been dried.
   Variation 3. Count out 100 kernels of punctured popcorn.
3. When it is your turn to use the popper, pop your kernels of corn for 2 minutes. Count the number of unpopped kernels that remain.
4. Write your results in your data table and on the board. In your data table, copy the results from the other variations.

Analyzing Results

1. Which variation had the smallest percentage of unpopped kernels? The largest percentage?

   _____
   _____

2. How do you explain these results?

   _____
   _____
   _____

(Continued on next page)

Food Science Lab Manual
Copyright © Mehas & Rodgers

EXPERIMENT 5-1 (Continued)

3. Does this one experiment prove your hypothesis is correct? Why or why not?
_____
_____
_____

4. How did you control the variables in this experiment?
_____
_____
_____

5. Based on your findings, how would you suggest storing popcorn to preserve its quality?
_____
_____
_____

6. Again based on these results, why do you think cracked kernels are discarded when popcorn is processed for sale?
_____
_____
_____

DATA TABLE

Variation	Number of Unpopped Kernels
Variation 1: unaltered popcorn	
Variation 2: dried popcorn	
Variation 3: punctured popcorn	

Name _____ Date _____ Class _____

Odor Recognition

EXPERIMENT 6-1

SAFETY FIRST
Review these safety guidelines before you begin this experiment.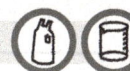

Normally, the senses of sight, odor, taste, touch, and, sometimes, hearing are used in evaluating food. When one sense is isolated, identification of even well-known samples can be difficult. This experiment will test your ability to identify common products by odor alone. Do not taste the samples.

Equipment and Materials
15 test tubes containing samples to be tested   test tube rack   blindfold

Procedure
1. From your teacher obtain 15 samples of odorous material, both food and nonfood, in coded test tubes.
2. Put on the blindfold. Sniff each of the 15 samples as your partner presents them for your evaluation. (Your partner should not sniff the samples while presenting them.) Your partner will record your identification of each sample in your data table.
3. Reverse roles, presenting each sample to your partner and recording his or her identifications.
4. Record the actual identification of each sample.

Analyzing Results

1. How many of the 15 substances did you identify correctly? How many did your partner identify?

   _____
   _____

2. Compare results to other class members. What were the highest and lowest number of correct identifications?

   _____
   _____

3. Which substances were the hardest and easiest to identify? Why?

   _____
   _____
   _____

(Continued on next page)

Food Science Lab Manual
Copyright © Mehas & Rodgers

EXPERIMENT 6-1 (Continued)

4. What does this experiment tell you about the interaction of the senses?

___
___
___

DATA TABLE

Substance Code Number	Your Identification	Actual Identity of Substance	Substance Code Number	Your Identification	Actual Identity of Substance

Name _____   Date _____ Class _____

Flavor Comparison

EXPERIMENT 6-2

SAFETY FIRST
Review these safety guidelines before you begin this experiment.

Tastes are divided into at least four categories: sweet, sour, bitter, or salty. In this experiment, you will compare the sweetness of common sugars and the tastes of sour and salty substances.

Equipment and Materials
5 sugar samples   5 sour samples   5 salty samples

Procedure

1. From your teacher, obtain small samples of the five sugars to be tested.
2. Taste each sample. (If you are diabetic, skip this part of the experiment. Continue with the other samples, ranking them as directed in Step 3 below.)
3. Compare each sample for sweetness. In your data table, rank the samples from least sweet (1) to most sweet (5).
4. Repeat Steps 1-3 with the sour samples.
5. Repeat Steps 1-3 with the salty samples.
6. Copy your rankings onto the board.
7. Copy the sample identifications provided by your teacher into your data table.

Analyzing Results

1. How do your rankings of the sugar samples compare with the class results? How do your rankings and the class rankings compare with the sweetness of sugars as listed in food science reference books?

_____
_____
_____
_____
_____

(Continued on next page)

Food Science Lab Manual
Copyright © Mehas & Rodgers

2. How do your findings on the sour samples compare with the class results? What relationship do you see between these rankings and the sour substances in the samples?

_____

_____

_____

3. Compare your results in the test of salty samples with the class results. How do your rankings and the class rankings compare with the amount of salts in each sample?

_____

_____

_____

4. Which group of samples did you have the most trouble ranking? Did the rest of the class have similar difficulty? Explain.

_____

_____

_____

_____

DATA TABLE

Rank	Sweet Samples		Sour Samples		Salty Samples	
	Sample Code	Identification	Sample Code	Identification	Sample Code	Identification
1						
2						
3						
4						
5						

Name _____ Date _____ Class _____

Mouthfeel and Sensory Evaluation

EXPERIMENT 6-3

SAFETY FIRST
Review these safety guidelines before you begin this experiment.

Mouthfeel is one of several sensations that contribute to the perception of flavor. Factors that influence mouthfeel include a food's shape, form, thickness, and temperature. Textural qualities, such as chewiness, brittleness, and density, also affect mouthfeel; so do hot or burning sensations due to spiciness or astringency (sourness).

In this experiment, you will study the impact of mouthfeel on your assessment of food. You will test samples with similar appearances, while holding your nose to eliminate odor as much as possible.

Equipment and Materials
4 food samples   paper towels   marking pen

Procedure
1. Obtain one sample of each of the four foods to be tested. Place each sample on a piece of paper towel. Mark the corresponding sample identification code on each piece of towel.
2. Offer the four samples to your lab partner, one at a time. Your partner should hold his or her nose. While chewing each sample, your partner should write the sample code in your data table and rate the sample on the traits listed there. Each trait should be rated high, low, or medium, depending on perception of that trait. The chosen response should be written in the appropriate space in your data table.
3. After tasting all four samples, your partner should repeat Steps 1 and 2 while you taste the samples and complete your data table.

Analyzing Results

1. What mouthfeel traits were most helpful in distinguishing among the four samples? The least useful?

_____
_____
_____
_____
_____
_____

(Continued on next page)

Food Science Lab Manual
Copyright © Mehas & Rodgers

EXPERIMENT 6-3 (Continued)

2. Could you detect odor even though you were holding your nose? Why or why not?

___

3. If asked to identify the samples, what would you say each one is?

___

DATA TABLE

Trait	Sample Code _____	Sample Code _____	Sample Code _____	Sample Code _____
Chewiness				
Astringency				
Thickness				
Graininess				
Brittleness				
Consistency				
Spiciness				

Name _____ Date _____ Class _____

EXPERIMENT 7-1
Separating Mixtures

SAFETY FIRST
Review these safety guidelines before you begin this experiment.

A mixture is composed of two or more substances that have not reacted with each other. The substances keep at least some of their original properties and can be separated by physical means.

In this experiment you'll mix known masses of sucrose (table sugar) and cornstarch and then add water to this mixture. One component of the mixture will dissolve in the water while the other won't. By filtering the mixture, you'll separate the component that doesn't dissolve (insoluble) from the other component. Drying the residue that is trapped on the filter paper as well as evaporating away the water that passes through the paper will allow you to recover both of the original solids.

Equipment and Materials

massing or waxed paper	2 beakers, 150-mL	filter paper	hotplate or burner
balance	water	funnel	beaker tongs
sucrose	100-mL graduated cylinder	ring stand with iron ring	paper
cornstarch	stirring rod	wash bottle	marking pen

Procedure

1. Using massing or waxed paper, mass between 1.0 and 1.5 g of sucrose and record the amount in your data table.
2. Repeat Step 1 using a second piece of massing paper and cornstarch.
3. Add both the sucrose and the cornstarch to a clean 150-mL beaker.
4. Using your 100-mL graduated cylinder, measure 30 mL of tap water and add to the beaker. Stir the mixture with a stirring rod to dissolve as much solid as possible.
5. Mass a piece of filter paper and record in your data table. Fold the filter paper in half, then in quarters. Open the folded paper to form a cone, with one thickness of paper on one side and three thicknesses on the other. Write your initials on the edge of the paper.
6. Place the paper in a funnel. Place the funnel in an iron ring that has been clamped to a ring stand. Moisten the filter paper with a small amount of water from a wash bottle.
7. Mass a second clean, dry, 150-mL beaker. Place this beaker under the funnel to catch the liquid that passes through the filter paper. (This liquid is called the filtrate.)
8. Decant (pour off) the liquid from the solid, leaving as much of the solid as possible in the beaker. Do this by pouring the liquid down a stirring rod into the funnel. Be careful to keep the liquid in the funnel below the top edge of the filter paper at all times. After nearly all the liquid has passed through the filter paper, use a stream of water from the wash bottle to wash all of the solid out of the beaker onto the filter paper.
9. After all the liquid has passed through the filter paper, wash the solid on the filter paper with more water from the wash bottle.
10. Carefully remove your filter paper from the funnel and place it on a tray designated by your teacher.
11. Heat the beaker containing the filtrate over medium heat until a solid begins to appear in the bottom of the beaker.

(Continued on next page)

Food Science Lab Manual
Copyright © Mehas & Rodgers

EXPERIMENT 7-1 (Continued)

12. Using beaker tongs, remove the beaker from the heat and place it on the lab table. Note the appearance of the contents of the beaker.
13. Place the beaker on a piece of paper with your initials on it on a second tray designated by your teacher.
14. The next day, mass the beaker and its contents, as well as the filter paper and the residue on it. Record these figures in your data table.
15. Subtract the mass of the beaker from the mass of beaker and contents. Subtract the mass of the filter paper from the mass of paper and residue. The remainder is the mass of sucrose and cornstarch recovered. Record these figures in your data table.

Analyzing Results

1. Which component of the original mixture dissolved in the water? Which one did not?

2. Were the sucrose and cornstarch completely separated by this procedure? Explain.

3. Did the sucrose have the same mass before and after the filtration process? Explain any difference.

4. Could you use this same procedure to separate sodium chloride (table salt) and sucrose? Explain.

DATA TABLE

Substance	Mass	Substance	Mass
Sucrose		Filter paper and residue	
Cornstarch		Residue	
Filter paper		Beaker and contents	
Beaker		Contents	

76

Food Science Lab Manual
Copyright © Mehas & Rodgers

Heterogeneous and Homogeneous Mixtures

EXPERIMENT 7-2

SAFETY FIRST
Review these safety guidelines before you begin this experiment.

In heterogeneous mixtures, individual ingredients can be visually recognized. In contrast, the substances present in homogeneous mixtures are evenly distributed so that the mixture appears to be a pure substance. This experiment will help you appreciate this difference in properties.

Equipment and Materials

250 g yogurt	100-mL graduated cylinder	1/2 banana
75 g strawberries	45 mL orange juice	40 g blueberries (optional)
10 g sugar	10-mL graduated cylinder	75 g pineapple (optional)
balance	7.0 mL vanilla	20-30 mL milk, if needed
blender	5-10 ice cubes	paper cup for each group member

Procedure

1. Mass 250 g yogurt, 75 g strawberries, and 10 g sugar. Put these ingredients in a blender.
2. Use a 100-mL graduated cylinder to measure 45 mL of orange juice. Add this to the ingredients in the blender.
3. Measure 7.0 mL of vanilla, using a 10-mL graduated cylinder. Add this to the blender.
4. Add 5-10 ice cubes, half a banana, and optional ingredients as desired to the blender.
5. Blend the mixture until smooth, about three minutes. If needed, add 20-30 mL milk to produce a beverage of drinking consistency.
6. Pour into paper cups and sample.

Analyzing Results

1. Was the drink a heterogeneous or a homogeneous mixture? Explain.

_____
_____
_____
_____
_____

(Continued on next page)

EXPERIMENT 7-2 (Continued)

2. Which ingredients are compounds?

   _____

   _____

   _____

3. Are the changes involved in preparing this drink physical or chemical changes? Explain.

   _____

   _____

   _____

Name _____ Date _____ Class _____

EXPERIMENT 7-3
The Boiling Point of Water

SAFETY FIRST
Review these safety guidelines before you begin this experiment.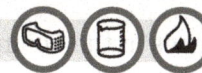

You may know from experience that it takes longer to boil a large amount of water than it does a small amount. Does this mean that the larger amount boils at a higher temperature? In this experiment, you will work to answer that question.

Equipment and Materials
250-mL beaker	ring stand	one-hole rubber stopper	safety goggles
thermometer	utility clamp	clock or watch with second hand	graph paper

Procedure

1. Pour the amount of water assigned by your teacher into a 250-mL beaker. Suspend a thermometer in the beaker, using a ring stand, utility clamp, and one-hole rubber stopper. In your data table, record the temperature of the liquid.
2. Heat the beaker of liquid on the range, reading and recording its temperature every 30 seconds. Wear safety goggles.
3. Continue to heat the liquid until about half of it has boiled away. Take readings the entire time the liquid is being heated.
4. Using graph paper, make a graph of your results. Plot the temperature of the liquid and the times at which your temperature readings were taken. Compare your results with those of classmates.

Analyzing Results

1. How do the graphs from different lab groups compare?

   _____

   _____

2. Do all graphs have a flat section, or plateau? If so, where?

   _____

   _____

3. At what temperature or temperatures did the liquid start to boil? _____

   _____

(Continued on next page)

EXPERIMENT 7-3 (Continued)

4. Was the temperature the same in all the beakers once the liquid started to boil?

   _____

   _____

5. How do you explain any differences in the boiling points recorded in different beakers?

   _____

   _____

   _____

6. Does the boiling point of pure water depend on the amount of water?

   _____

   _____

   _____

DATA TABLE

Time	Temperature	Time	Temperature

Physical Changes and Chemical Reactions

EXPERIMENT 8-1

SAFETY FIRST
Review these safety guidelines before you begin this experiment.

When matter undergoes a physical change, only size, shape, temperature, or physical state of the substance alters. Examples of physical changes are freezing or melting, boiling or condensing, dissolving, grinding, tearing, and breaking into smaller pieces. Physical changes produce no new substances. On the other hand, one or more new substances always result during chemical reactions.

In this experiment you will cause several substances to undergo change. By observing the products, you'll determine whether a physical change or a chemical reaction occurred.

Equipment and Materials

iron filings (Fe)	paper	stirring rod	watch glass
sodium hydrogen carbonate ($NaHCO_3$)	magnet	ring stand	safety goggles
	spatula	iron ring	hotplate or burner
sodium chloride (NaCl)	6 test tubes	funnel	crucible tongs or forceps
sucrose ($C_{12}H_{22}O_{11}$)	test tube rack	filter paper	beaker tongs
sand (SiO_2)	water	wash bottle	3 mL vinegar
magnifying glass	3 beakers, 150-mL		

Procedure: Part I

1. Place small samples of each of the five solids (Fe, $NaHCO_3$, NaCl, $C_{12}H_{22}O_{11}$, SiO_2) on a piece of paper. Examine each with a magnifying glass. Record your observations in Data Table A.
2. Test the effect of a magnet on each substance by lifting the paper and passing the magnet under it.
3. Test solubility by placing half of each sample in a clean, dry test tube and adding 5 mL of water. Tap the side of the tube with your finger to mix the solid and water completely.

Procedure: Part II

4. Mix the remaining iron filings with the sand on a single piece of paper. Test with the magnet as before.
5. Transfer the mixture of iron filings and sand, along with the remaining sodium chloride, to a clean 150-mL beaker. Add 30 mL of water and stir. Record your observations in Data Table B.
6. Attach an iron ring to a ring stand. Place a funnel in the iron ring. Fold a piece of filter paper in half, and then in half again to form a cone. Open the cone so that three layers of paper are on one side, and one layer is on the other. Place the paper in the funnel. Moisten it slightly with water from a wash bottle to hold it in place. Place a second 150-mL beaker under the funnel to catch the filtrate (the liquid passing through the filter paper).
7. Decant (pour off) the liquid from the solid by pouring it down a stirring rod into the funnel. Be careful to keep the liquid below the top edge of the filter paper at all times. After nearly all the liquid has passed through the filter paper, use a stream of water from the wash bottle to wash all of the solid out of the beaker onto the filter paper.
8. After all the liquid has passed through the filter paper, wash the solid on the filter paper with more water from the wash bottle.

(Continued on next page)

Food Science Lab Manual
Copyright © Mehas & Rodgers

EXPERIMENT 8-1 (Continued)

9. Examine the solid remaining on the filter paper. Record your observations in Data Table B. Set the filter paper aside for later examination.
10. Pour a small amount of the filtrate onto a watch glass. Put on safety goggles. Heat the watch glass over medium heat on a hotplate or burner until the liquid has completely evaporated. Remove the watch glass from the heat, using crucible tongs or forceps. With the magnifying glass, examine the solid remaining and describe it in Data Table B.
11. Place the remaining sucrose in a clean, dry 150-mL beaker. Place it over medium heat, noting any changes in appearance. Every two or three minutes remove the beaker from the heat, using beaker tongs, and check for odors by fanning the fumes toward your nose. Place the beaker over high heat for 1 to 2 minutes longer. Remove it from the heat and allow it to cool to room temperature.
12. Carefully unfold the filter paper reserved in Step 9. Spread out the residue on the paper with the stirring rod. Pass the magnet under the paper and record what you observe in Data Table B.
13. After the beaker used to heat the sugar has cooled to room temperature, examine the solid remaining in the beaker. Add a few milliliters of water to test its solubility.
14. Add the remaining sodium hydrogen carbonate to a clean, dry test tube and add 3 mL of vinegar. Feel the bottom of the test tube. Record your observations.
15. Follow your teacher's instructions for proper disposal of materials.

Analyzing Results

1. Did the properties of any of the substances change when they were mixed on the paper with other substances?

___

2. Was dissolving the substances in water a physical or chemical change? How do you know?

___

3. Did heating produce a physical or chemical change in the filtrate? In the sugar?

___

(Continued on next page)

Name _____ Date _____ Class _____

EXPERIMENT 8-1 (Continued)

4. Was dissolving the sodium hydrogen carbonate in the vinegar a physical or a chemical change? How do you know?

_____

_____

_____

_____

DATA TABLE A

Substance	Formula	Color	Effect of Magnet	Solubility in Water
Iron filings				
Sodium hydrogen carbonate				
Sodium chloride				
Sucrose				
Sand				

(Continued on next page)

EXPERIMENT 8-1 (Continued)

DATA TABLE B

Substance	Observations
Iron and sand mixture	
Iron, sand, and salt mixed with water	
Residue (solid) on filter paper	
Solid remaining after evaporation of filtrate	
Sugar heated	
Sodium hydrogen carbonate with vinegar	

Name _____ Date _____ Class _____

Changes Involved in Making Peanut Brittle

EXPERIMENT 8-2

SAFETY FIRST
Review these safety guidelines before you begin this experiment.

A phase change is only a physical change: the material remains the same substance. Likewise, when materials are simply mixed together, only a physical change occurs. The original materials are still present, but no longer in a pure form. If a chemical change occurs, however, new materials with different chemical properties are produced. This change usually cannot be reversed.

In this experiment you will observe the physical and chemical changes that occur in the process of making peanut brittle.

Equipment and Materials

225 g sugar	cookie sheet	candy thermometer	100 g peanuts
0.5 g baking soda	aluminum foil	burner or hotplate	(chopped if desired)
10 g margarine	saucepan	spoon	

Procedure

1. Mass the sugar, baking soda, and margarine. Assemble them for use, as you will need to mix them quickly.
2. Cover a cookie sheet with aluminum foil.
3. Place the sugar in a saucepan over medium heat for about 2 minutes or until all of the sugar has become liquid. Using a candy thermometer, measure the temperature of the liquid and record it.
4. Add the baking soda and the margarine. Stir quickly until mixed. Add the peanuts.
5. Spread the mixture on the foil-covered cookie sheet.
6. Let cool; then break the mixture into 2- to 3-cm pieces.

Analyzing Results

1. Describe any change of state that you observed.

_____
_____
_____
_____

(Continued on next page)

Food Science Lab Manual
Copyright © Mehas & Rodgers

EXPERIMENT 8-2 (Continued)

2. Describe any chemical changes that took place. What evidence do you have that these were chemical changes?

   _____
   _____
   _____

3. If chopped, did the peanuts undergo a physical or a chemical change? Why?

   _____
   _____
   _____

4. Was the liquefying of the sugar a physical or a chemical change? Why?

   _____
   _____
   _____

5. What is the melting point of sugar? How do you know?

   _____
   _____
   _____

6. Why did the mixture prepared in the saucepan become a solid?

   _____
   _____
   _____

7. When did the brittle change from a homogeneous to a heterogeneous mixture? Why?

   _____
   _____
   _____

Name _____ Date _____ Class _____

Boiling Points of Sugar and Salt Solutions

EXPERIMENT 8-3

SAFETY FIRST
Review these safety guidelines before you begin this experiment.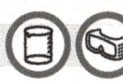

The boiling point of a solution varies with concentration. As a solution boils, water evaporates, and the solution becomes more concentrated. In this experiment, you will observe sugar and salt solutions during heating to determine how the presence of a solute, and its concentration, affect the boiling point of water.

Equipment and Materials

sugar or salt solution
250-mL beaker
candy thermometer
ring stand
utility clamp
one-hole rubber stopper
safety goggles
clock or watch with second hand
graph paper

Procedure

1. Pour 150 mL of the solution provided by your teacher into a 250-mL beaker. Suspend a thermometer in the beaker, using a ring stand, utility clamp, and one-hole rubber stopper. Record the temperature of the liquid in your data table.
2. Heat the solution, reading and recording the temperature of the liquid every 30 seconds. Wear safety goggles throughout the heating process. Note in your data table the temperature at which the liquid reaches a full rolling boil.
3. Continue to heat the solution for 15 minutes, or until about half the liquid has boiled away, whichever comes first. Continue to take readings every 30 seconds the entire time the liquid is being heated. Expand your data table on separate paper if needed.
4. Record any change in appearance of the solution as heating proceeds.
5. Using graph paper, make a graph of your results. Plot the temperature of the liquid and the times at which your temperature readings were taken. Compare your results with those of your classmates, and with your graph from Experiment 7-3, The Boiling Point of Water.

Analyzing Results

1. How does the temperature at which your solution boiled compare with the boiling point of pure water, as you recorded in Experiment 7-3?

_____

_____

_____

(Continued on next page)

Food Science Lab Manual
Copyright © Mehas & Rodgers

2. Did your solution boil at a constant temperature? If not, how did the boiling point change? How do you account for this change?

_____
_____
_____

3. If the boiling point remained constant, what would explain this?

_____
_____
_____

4. Compare the graphs of the sugar and the salt solutions. What would explain any differences you observe?

_____
_____
_____
_____

5. What can you conclude about the relationship between the boiling point of water and the boiling point of a water solution? Between the boiling point of a solution and its concentration?

_____
_____
_____

DATA TABLE
Type of Solution _____

Time	Temperature	Change in Appearance	Time	Temperature	Change in Appearance

Food Science Lab Manual
Copyright © Mehas & Rodgers

The Solvent Properties of Water

EXPERIMENT 9-1

SAFETY FIRST
Review these safety guidelines before you begin this experiment.

Water is a very effective solvent for a variety of solutes. In this experiment you will compare the solvent properties of water to those of two other household liquids. **Note**: Alcohol is a flammable liquid. Keep it away from flames.

Equipment and Materials
10-mL graduated cylinder	balance	6.0 g sucrose
water	stirring rod	25.0 mL rubbing alcohol
8 test tubes	6.0 g sodium chloride	25.0 mL vegetable oil
test tube rack		

Procedure
1. Using the 10-mL graduated cylinder, measure and add 10 mL of water to each of four clean test tubes in a test tube rack.
2. Mass 2.0 g of sodium chloride and add to the first test tube. Stir with a clean stirring rod and record your observations in your data table.
3. Mass 2.0 g of sucrose and add to the second test tube. Stir with a clean stirring rod and record your observations.
4. Measure 5.0 mL of rubbing alcohol with the 10-mL graduated cylinder. Add this to the water in the third test tube. Stir with a clean stirring rod and record your observations.
5. Measure 5.0 mL of vegetable oil with the 10-mL graduated cylinder. Add this to the water in the fourth test tube. Stir with a clean stirring rod and record your observations.
6. Using the 10-mL graduated cylinder, measure and add 10 mL of alcohol to each of two clean test tubes.
7. Add 2.0 g of sodium chloride to one test tube of alcohol, and 2.0 g of sucrose to the other. Record your observations in your data table.
8. Add 10 mL of vegetable oil to each of two additional, clean test tubes.
9. Add 2.0 g of sodium chloride to one test tube of vegetable oil, and 2.0 g of sucrose to the other. Record your observations in your data table.

Analyzing Results
1. Which liquid dissolved the two solids completely?

_____

2. Which liquid or liquids dissolved in water?

_____

(Continued on next page)

Food Science Lab Manual
Copyright © Mehas & Rodgers

EXPERIMENT 9-1 (Continued)

3. Given that water is a polar molecule, alcohol is a slightly polar molecule, and vegetable oil is nonpolar, explain your answer to the second question.

_____

_____

_____

_____

4. Again remembering their relative polarities, explain each liquid's ability or inability to dissolve sodium chloride, an ionic compound, and sucrose, a polar molecular substance.

_____

_____

_____

_____

DATA TABLE

Mixture	Behavior
Sodium chloride in water	
Sucrose in water	
Alcohol in water	
Vegetable oil in water	
Sodium chloride in alcohol	
Sucrose in alcohol	
Sodium chloride in vegetable oil	
Sucrose in vegetable oil	

Name _____ Date _____ Class _____

Purifying Water

EXPERIMENT 9-2

SAFETY FIRST
Review these safety guidelines before you begin this experiment.

In many parts of the United States, chlorine is added to water to make this essential nutrient safe for consumption. In this experiment, you will observe the effect of chlorine on living organisms found in pond water. The source of chlorine will be household bleach.

Equipment and Materials
- 20 mL pond water
- 25-mL graduated cylinder
- 10-mL graduated cylinder
- 2 test tubes
- test-tube rack
- 10 mL chlorine bleach
- test tube stopper
- dropper
- microscope slide
- microscope
- plastic squeeze bottle

Procedure
1. Obtain 20 mL of pond water in a 25-mL graduated cylinder. Pour 10 mL of this water into one test tube and 10 mL into a second test tube.
2. Add 10 mL of chlorine bleach to one of the test tubes. Stopper the test tube and shake well.
3. With a dropper, place a few drops of the untreated water on a microscope slide and observe it under the microscope. Record your observations in your data table.
4. Thoroughly wash the dropper and slide. Then repeat Step 3 using a few drops of the treated water.

Analyzing Results
1. What effect did the chlorine bleach have on the organisms present?

_____
_____
_____
_____

(Continued on next page)

Food Science Lab Manual
Copyright © Mehas & Rodgers

EXPERIMENT 9-2 (Continued)

2. Chlorine bleach is often recommended for disinfecting cutting boards. How is this related to the effect of chlorine on the pond water?

_____

_____

_____

3. Does your local water supply contain chlorine? If so, in what ratio? (Contact your water district to find out.)

_____

_____

_____

DATA TABLE

Sample	Observations
Untreated water	
Treated water	

Name _____ Date _____ Class _____

EXPERIMENT 9-3
Bottled Water Taste Test

SAFETY FIRST
Review these safety guidelines before you begin this experiment.

Bottled water has become increasingly popular in recent years. Some prefer the taste of bottled water to their local tap water. Others choose to drink bottled water rather than carbonated beverages containing sugar or sugar substitutes. In this experiment you will use the some of the sensory evaluation techniques you learned in Chapter 6 to conduct a taste test of six brands of bottled water.

Equipment and Materials
numbered bottles containing six brands of bottled water   paper cup

Procedure
1. Pour approximately 50 mL of one of the bottled water samples into a paper cup.
2. Identify the sample by number in your data table.
3. Taste the sample and rate it on each quality in your data table. Use a scale from 1 (agreeable) to 5 (disagreeable).
4. Repeat with the other five brands, rinsing your cup with tap water between each test.
5. Add your ratings for each sample. Record that overall score in your data table. (The lowest score indicates your favorite.)
6. After students have completed taste-testing the samples and have filled in their data tables, your teacher will identify the samples by brand name.

Analyzing Results
1. Which quality did you find most influenced your ratings of the bottled water?
   _____

2. Which qualities were hardest to evaluate individually? Why do you think this was so?
   _____
   _____
   _____
   _____
   _____

(Continued on next page)

Food Science Lab Manual
Copyright © Mehas & Rodgers

EXPERIMENT 9-3 (Continued)

3. If you drink bottled water regularly, was the brand you chose as your favorite in the taste test the same brand that you buy? If not, in what ways was the favorite brand superior?

___

___

___

___

DATA TABLE

Sample No.	Flavor	Aftertaste	Carbonation	Overall Score	Brand Name

Name _____ Date _____ Class _____

EXPERIMENT 10-1
Neutralization

SAFETY FIRST
Review these safety guidelines before you begin this experiment.

In this experiment, you'll compare the acetic acid content of several brands of vinegar by titrating equal volumes of the vinegar with the base sodium hydroxide (NaOH). You'll determine how much base is needed to neutralize the acid in the vinegar. The more acid present, the more base you will need to neutralize it.

Equipment and Materials
safety goggles
2 burets, 50-mL
2 ring stands
2 utility clamps
1.0-M sodium hydroxide (NaOH) solution
vinegar sample (one brand)
250-mL Erlenmeyer flask
phenolphthalein solution

Procedure
1. Put on safety goggles and wear them throughout this experiment. NaOH can harm the eyes.
2. Clamp two clean, 50-mL burets to ring stands. Fill one buret with 1.0-M NaOH solution.
3. Fill the second buret with the brand of vinegar assigned by your teacher.
4. Add 20 mL of vinegar from the buret to a clean, 250-mL Erlenmeyer flask. Add three drops of the indicator phenolphthalein to the vinegar. Place the flask under the tip of the buret containing the NaOH.
5. Slowly add the NaOH to the vinegar. A pink color appears where the base first contacts the acid. Gently swirl the flask until the color disappears. Add the base drop by drop, swirling after each drop, until the base turns the solution to a pale pink that does not disappear.
6. In your data table, record the volume of NaOH used.
7. Wash out the flask and repeat the titration. If you used more than 25 mL of base, be sure to refill the buret before beginning the second titration.
8. Again record the volume of base required. Average the two amounts and record.
9. Report your figures on the board.
10. In your data table, record the figures for each of the brands of vinegar tested by the other experiment groups.

Analyzing Results
1. What observation can you make about the amount of acetic acid in the various brands of vinegar? How do you explain this?

_____
_____
_____
_____

(Continued on next page)

EXPERIMENT 10-1 (Continued)

2. What was the function of the indicator in this experiment?

　_____

　_____

3. Would you use the same vinegar for pickling, where very low pH is important, as you would in a salad? Why or why not?

　_____

　_____

　_____

DATA TABLE

Brand of Vinegar	Volume of Base		
	Trial 1	Trial 2	Average

Name _____ Date _____ Class _____

The pH of Common Foods

EXPERIMENT 10-2

SAFETY FIRST
Review these safety guidelines before you begin this experiment.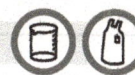

The pH of food is important for several reasons. How acidic or basic a food is influences its taste. Acidic pH values tend to prevent food from spoiling. In this experiment, you will test some common foods and food ingredients to determine their pH values.

Equipment and Materials

14 test tubes masking tape pH indicator paper deionized water
test tube rack marking pen tap water all foods and food ingredients listed in table

Procedure

1. Working with another lab group, prepare half a test tube of each of the items in your data table. Follow the descriptions provided in the table. Shake any mixtures to be sure they are dissolved. Label each test tube with the name of the contents.
2. Using pH indicator paper, determine the pH of each solution by dipping the paper into each liquid sample and matching the color to the chart provided. In your data table, record your results.
3. After the pH of all 14 substances has been tested, combine the contents of test tubes 3 and 4. Mix thoroughly. Record the pH of the resulting solution.

Analyzing Results

1. Based on pH, categorize the solutions as acidic, basic, or neutral.

_____

_____

_____

_____

2. What pH resulted from mixing test tubes 3 and 4? How do you explain this result?

_____

_____

_____

_____

(Continued on next page)

Food Science Lab Manual
Copyright © Mehas & Rodgers

EXPERIMENT 10-2 (Continued)

3. What did you observe when you mixed test tubes 3 and 4? How is this chemical reaction used in preparing some foods?

_____

_____

_____

4. Do you think all tap water has the same pH? Why or why not?

_____

_____

_____

DATA TABLE

Test Tube Number	Solution	pH
1	Tap water	
2	Deionized water	
3	Vinegar (5% acetic acid)	
4	Sodium bicarbonate (a few crystals) dissolved in deionized water	
5	Egg white	
6	5 mL honey dissolved in tap water	
7	5 mL molasses dissolved in tap water	
8	Buttermilk	
9	Lemon juice	
10	Cream of tartar (a few grains) dissolved in tap water	
11	Lemon-lime soda	
12	Cranberry-apple juice	
13	Milk	
14	Powdered orange drink dissolved in tap water	
3-4	Mixture of test tubes 3 and 4	

Red Cabbage Juice Indicator

EXPERIMENT 10-3

SAFETY FIRST
Review these safety guidelines before you begin this experiment.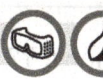

In addition to commercially prepared chemical indicators, many plant pigments change color when they are mixed with acids or bases. In this experiment, you will prepare an indicator from red cabbage and observe its behavior when mixed with known acids and bases. You will then use the indicator to discover whether two unknown solutions are acidic or basic.

Equipment and Materials

red cabbage	safety goggles	all foods and food ingredients listed in table
knife	7 test tubes and rack	dropper
400-mL beaker	10-mL graduated cylinder	

Procedure

1. In your data table record the pH of the five known items listed. Refer to the results from Experiment 10-2, The pH of Common Foods, for this information.
2. Place several pieces of red cabbage in a 400-mL beaker. Add just enough tap water to cover the cabbage. After putting on safety goggles, heat the water to boiling. Boil several minutes until the liquid turns a dark purple. You may remove your safety goggles after you have finished heating the solution.
3. Place 5 mL of the first solution to be tested in a test tube. Use a dropper to add 10 drops of the cabbage indicator to the test tube. Record the indicator color in your data table.
4. Repeat Steps 2-3 with the other known items listed in your data table.
5. Obtain 5 mL of unknown X and place in a test tube. Add 10 drops of the cabbage indicator to the test tube. In your data table, record the color of the indicator, and, if possible, an approximate pH value.
6. Repeat Step 5 with unknown Y.
7. Pour the unknown solutions together and note the color of the mixture. If possible, estimate the pH of the mixture. Record this information in your data table.

(Continued on next page)

Food Science Lab Manual
Copyright © Mehas & Rodgers

EXPERIMENT 10-3 (Continued)

Analyzing Results

1. What color does the cabbage indicator turn in an acid? In a base?

   Acid: _____   Base: _____

2. Was unknown X an acid or a base? Unknown Y?

   X: _____   Y: _____

3. Based on the appearance of the mixture when the two unknowns were combined, which was stronger, unknown X or unknown Y? How do you know this?

   _____
   _____
   _____

DATA TABLE

Solution	pH	Color of Indicator
Vinegar		
Lemon-lime soda		
Tap water		
Sodium bicarbonate		
Egg white		
Unknown X		
Unknown Y		
Mixed unknowns		

Name _____ Date _____ Class _____

Effect of Surface Area on Cooking Rate

EXPERIMENT 11-1

SAFETY FIRST
Review these safety guidelines before you begin this experiment.

In this experiment, you will use different-sized pieces of potato to study the effect of surface area on cooking rate.

Equipment and Materials

100-mL graduated cylinder
400-mL beaker
potato
paring knife
2.5-cm square, cut from an index card
wooden toothpicks

Procedure

1. Measure 200 mL of water using the 100-mL graduated cylinder. Pour the water into a 400-mL beaker. Place over medium-high heat on a range burner.
2. While the water is heating, obtain a potato from your teacher. From the potato, cut a cube measuring 2.5 cm on each side. Use the index card square as a guide for cutting to size.
3. Follow one of the following variations as assigned by your teacher:
   Variation 1. Use the single cube of potato.
   Variation 2. Cut the cube into 8 equal-size cubes by cutting the original cube in half in all three directions.
   Variation 3. Cut the cube into 27 equal-size cubes by cutting the original cube in thirds in all three directions.
4. Place the potato cube or cubes in the water after it has come to a boil.
5. At 1-minute intervals, test the potato with a wooden toothpick. Based on how easily the toothpick punctures the potato, determine its degree of doneness, for example, uncooked, slightly cooked, cooked. Record this information in your data table.
6. When the toothpick punctures the potato easily, note the time in your data table. Turn off the burner and remove the beaker from the range.
7. On the board, record the number of the variation you followed and the time needed to cook the potato.

(Continued on next page)

Food Science Lab Manual
Copyright © Mehas & Rodgers

EXPERIMENT 11-1 (Continued)

Analyzing Results

1. Was there a difference in the total volume of potato present in each beaker?

   _____

2. Was there any relationship between the size of the potato cubes and their cooking time? If so, describe it.

   _____

   _____

   _____

3. Explain the difference in cooking time.

   _____

   _____

DATA TABLE
Variation Number _____

Time in Minutes	Degree of Doneness	Time in Minutes	Degree of Doneness

Name _____ Date _____ Class _____

Effect of Temperature on Cooking Rate

EXPERIMENT 11-2

SAFETY FIRST
Review these safety guidelines before you begin this experiment.

In this experiment, you will study the effect of temperature on the cooking rate of food—in this case, a potato.

Equipment and Materials

potato	400-mL beaker	one-hole stopper
2.5-cm square from index card	thermometer	safety goggles
paring knife	ring stand	tongs or slotted spoon
100-mL graduated cylinder	utility clamp	wooden toothpick

Procedure

1. Obtain a potato from your teacher. From the potato, cut a cube measuring 2.5 cm on each side. Use a 2.5-cm square cut from an index card as a cutting guide.
2. Measure 200 mL of water, using a 100-mL graduated cylinder. Pour the water into a 400-mL beaker. The water should be deep enough to completely immerse the cube of potato, which will be added later.
3. Suspend a thermometer in the beaker, using a ring stand, utility clamp, and one-hole stopper. Then follow the variation assigned by your teacher. Wear safety goggles throughout the heating process.
   Variation 1. Heat the water to 90°C.
   Variation 2. Heat the water to 100°C.
4. Monitor the water temperature, removing the beaker or turning down the heat as necessary to keep the temperature constant.
5. When you can keep the water temperature constant, immerse the potato cube in the water.
6. Cook the potato. Remove it from the water every 2 minutes with tongs or a slotted spoon. Test the potato quickly by puncturing with a wooden toothpick and return the potato immediately to the water. Based on how easily the toothpick punctures the potato, determine its degree of doneness; for example, uncooked, slightly cooked, cooked. Record this information in your data table. Expand the table on separate paper if needed.
7. When the toothpick punctures the potato easily, note the time in your data table. Turn off the heat and remove the beaker from the range.
8. On the board, record your variation number and the time needed to cook the potato.
9. List the times required to cook each of the potato cubes that were in the 90°C water. Make a similar list for the potato cubes in 100°C water.

(Continued on next page)

Food Science Lab Manual
Copyright © Mehas & Rodgers

EXPERIMENT 11-2 (Continued)

Analyzing Results

1. What is the average cooking time for the potato cubes in the 90°C water? For the potato cubes in 100°C water?

   _____

   _____

2. What is the difference in average cooking times for the two temperatures? How do you explain this difference?

   _____

   _____

   _____

3. How can you use what you have learned from this experiment to help in preparing food?

   _____

   _____

   _____

DATA TABLE

Your Test at _____ °C		Class Cooking Times at 90°C	Class Cooking Times at 100°C
Time in Minutes	Degree of Doneness		

Heat Transfer Through Metal

EXPERIMENT 11-3

SAFETY FIRST
Review these safety guidelines before you begin this experiment.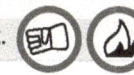

Heat transfer through cookware takes place when food is cooked on a surface heating element on a range. To promote even cooking, the materials used to make cookware need to conduct heat rapidly and uniformly. In this experiment, you will test several frying pans to discover which ones conduct heat the most quickly and evenly.

Equipment and Materials
frying pans made of different metals   oil   flour

Procedure

1. Make sure the frying pan you're testing isn't hot. Lightly grease and flour the pan. Remove any excess flour by turning the pan upside down over the sink and tapping the bottom with the flat of your hand.
2. On medium heat, preheat the large heating element on the range for 2 minutes. Use the same burner on the same setting for each pan tested.
3. Place the pan on the burner and time how long it takes for the flour coating to turn a light golden brown.
4. In your data table, identify the pan by its metal composition. Record the time needed for browning to occur. Note whether the flour coating is evenly browned or browned only in spots. Record these observations in your data table.
5. When the pan is cool, thoroughly wash and dry it.
6. Repeat Steps 1-5 with each pan to be tested. If necessary, trade pans with other lab groups until you have tested all the pans specified by your teacher.

Analyzing Results

1. Which pan heated the most quickly?

   _____

   _____

2. Which pan conducted heat most evenly?

   _____

   _____

   _____

(Continued on next page)

Food Science Lab Manual
Copyright © Mehas & Rodgers

EXPERIMENT 11-3 (Continued)

3. Which do you think is the best pan to use for cooking? Why?

   _____

   _____

4. What might explain the differences in heating times and evenness among different pans?

   _____

   _____

   _____

   _____

DATA TABLE

Frying Pan Type	Browning Time	Evenness of Browning

Name _____   Date _____ Class _____

Identifying Basic Nutrients in Foods

EXPERIMENT 12-1

SAFETY FIRST
Review these safety guidelines before you begin this experiment.

In this experiment you will test for the presence of complex carbohydrates (starch), simple carbohydrates (sugar), fats, and proteins in several common foods.

Equipment and Materials

5 test tubes	iodine solution	egg albumin
test tube rack	Benedict's solution	bread suspension
10-mL graduated cylinder	burner or hotplate	banana suspension
400-mL beaker	Biuret reagent	fat-free milk
metric ruler	starch suspension	whole milk
safety goggles	dextrose solution	potato suspension
brown paper	vegetable oil	

Procedure: Part I

1. Place four clean test tubes in a test tube rack. Add 3 mL of starch solution to test tube 1; 3 mL of dextrose solution to test tube 2; 3 mL of egg albumin (protein) to test tube 3; and 3 mL of water into test tube 4.
2. To each of these test tubes add one drop of dilute iodine solution. Record any color change in your data table.
3. Wash the test tubes. Then repeat Step 1.
4. To each of the test tubes, add 5 mL of Benedict's solution. Place the test tubes in a 400-mL beaker containing enough water to completely surround the liquid in the test tubes. Wearing safety goggles, heat the water in the beaker to boiling; and then boil for three minutes. Record any color change you observe in your data table.
5. Again wash and then prepare the test tubes as in Step 1.
6. Add 3 mL of water to each of the four test tubes.
7. Wear safety goggles as you add 5 drops of Biuret reagent to all four test tubes. Be careful not to get this solution on your hands. If any should contact your skin, wash it off immediately using plenty of water. Record any color change you observe in your data table.
8. Since fats don't dissolve in water, a different type of test is needed to check for their presence. Place a drop of the starch, dextrose, and protein solutions, plus a drop of vegetable oil (fat) on a piece of brown paper. Hold the paper up to a light. Any sample containing fat will produce a translucent spot on the paper. Describe the appearance of the paper in your data table.

(Continued on next page)

Food Science Lab Manual
Copyright © Mehas & Rodgers

107

EXPERIMENT 12-1 (Continued)

Procedure: Part II

9. Place 5 clean test tubes in your test tube rack. Obtain 3-mL samples of the suspensions of bread, banana, and potato flakes prepared by your teacher. Also obtain 3-mL samples of fat-free and whole milk. Place these in the test tubes. Test with iodine as in Step 2 and record results in your data table.
10. Wash and then prepare test tubes as in Step 9, then test each sample with Benedict's solution as you did in Step 4. Record results in your data table.
11. Wash and again prepare test tubes as in Step 9, and test each sample with Biuret reagent as in Step 7. Remember to keep your safety goggles on whenever using Biuret reagent. Record your results in your data table.
12. Place a small amount of each of the five foods being tested on a piece of brown paper as in Step 8, to test for the presence of fat.

Analyzing Results

1. With what type of nutrient did each reagent react? What color changes indicated this?

_____
_____
_____

2. What can you conclude about the nutrient content of each food tested?

_____
_____
_____
_____
_____

3. Did any of the foods seem to contain only one type of nutrient? If so, explain.

_____
_____
_____
_____

4. How do whole milk and fat-free milk differ in nutrient content?

_____
_____
_____

(Continued on next page)

Name _____ Date _____ Class _____

EXPERIMENT 12-1 (Continued)

DATA TABLE: Part A

Nutrient Tested	Reagent Used			
	Iodine Solution	Benedict's Solution	Biuret Reagent	Brown Paper
Starch				
Sugar				
Protein				
Water				
Fat				

DATA TABLE: Part B

Food Tested	Reagent Used			
	Iodine Solution	Benedict's Solution	Biuret Reagent	Brown Paper
Bread				
Banana				
Potato flakes				
Whole milk				
Fat-Free milk				

Food Science Lab Manual
Copyright © Mehas & Rodgers

Calcium in Milk

EXPERIMENT 12-2

SAFETY FIRST
Review these safety guidelines before you begin this experiment.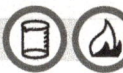

The enzyme rennin causes milk to coagulate by converting the milk protein casein into a compound called paracasein. For rennin to work, however, calcium ions must be present. When calcium ions are removed from milk, coagulation is suppressed. In this experiment, you will observe the effects of calcium ions on the coagulation of milk.

Equipment and Materials

3 test tubes	400-mL beaker	rennet	dropper
whole milk	thermometer	sodium citrate	calcium chloride
labels or grease pencil	balance	3 rubber stoppers	

Procedure

1. Fill three test tubes three-fourths full of whole milk. Label them A, B, and C.
2. Heat water in a 400-mL beaker to a temperature of 37°C. Place all three test tubes in the water. Maintain heat at 37°C.
3. Add 0.1 g of rennet, a substance that contains the enzyme rennin, to tube A. Add 0.1 g of rennet and 0.1 g of sodium citrate to tube B. This compound reacts with calcium ions to make them unavailable to react with the rennin. Tube C will be the control in the experiment, the standard with which other samples are compared.
4. Stopper the tubes. Allow them to sit for 5 minutes in the water bath.
5. Examine the contents of the test tubes. Turn them upside down, but do not shake them. Record your observations in your data table.
6. Add 4-5 drops of calcium chloride solution to tube B. Replace it in the water bath with the other tubes for an additional 5 minutes. Again, record your observations in your data table.

Analyzing Results

1. Compare test tube A with test tube C. How do they differ?

_____

_____

_____

_____

(Continued on next page)

EXPERIMENT 12-2 (Continued)

2. How did the milk in test tube B respond to the addition of rennet and sodium citrate? To the addition of calcium chloride?

   _____

   _____

   _____

3. How do you explain the observations you described in question 2?

   _____

   _____

   _____

   _____

4. Why do you think the milk was placed in a water bath for this experiment?

   _____

   _____

   _____

DATA TABLE

Test Tube	Appearance After 5 Minutes	Appearance After 10 Minutes
A		
B		
C		

Name _____ Date _____ Class _____

Nutrition Facts Panel

EXPERIMENT 12-3

SAFETY FIRST
Review these safety guidelines before you begin this experiment.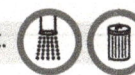

The Nutrition Facts panel on food packaging tells the consumer what nutrients are present in the food and what percent of the recommended Daily Value of that nutrient the food provides. This gives consumers a general idea about how much of their overall daily nutrient intake is provided by the food in question.

In this experiment you will compare labels for three brands each of peanut butter, jam or jelly, and bread in order to decide which combination will provide you with the most nutritious sandwich.

Equipment and Materials
9 Nutrition Facts panels

Procedure
1. Examine the Nutrition Facts panels on the peanut butter, jelly, and bread labels provided by your teacher.
2. Record the information required in your data table.

Analyzing Results

1. Which peanut butter is highest in calories? Highest in saturated fat?

   _____
   _____

2. Is the peanut butter with the highest saturated fat content also the one with the highest calorie content?

   _____
   _____

3. Which bread do you think has the highest overall nutritional value? Why?

   _____
   _____
   _____

(Continued on next page)

Food Science Lab Manual
Copyright © Mehas & Rodgers

EXPERIMENT 12-3 (Continued)

4. Which combination of peanut butter, jelly, and bread would provide you with the lowest calorie sandwich?
   _____
   _____

5. Which combination would be:
   a. highest in fiber? _____
   b. lowest in saturated fat? _____
   c. lowest in sugar? _____
   d. highest in iron? _____

6. Which combination of peanut butter, jelly, and bread offers the most nutritious sandwich? Why?
   _____
   _____
   _____
   _____

7. Which combination do you think would be the most tasty? Why?
   _____
   _____
   _____

8. If your answers to questions 6 and 7 are not the same, which combination of products would you use for your sandwich? Why?
   _____
   _____
   _____
   _____

(Continued on next page)

Name _____ Date _____ Class _____

EXPERIMENT 12-3 (Continued)

DATA TABLE

Label Information	Peanut Butter A	Peanut Butter B	Peanut Butter C	Jam or Jelly D	Jam or Jelly E	Jam or Jelly F	Bread G	Bread H	Bread I
Serving size									
Calories									
Total fat									
Saturated fat									
Cholesterol									
Sodium									
Total carbohydrate									
Dietary fiber									
Sugars									
Protein									
Vitamin A									
Vitamin C									
Calcium									
Iron									

Food Science Lab Manual
Copyright © Mehas & Rodgers

Digestion of Starch

EXPERIMENT 13-1

SAFETY FIRST
Review these safety guidelines before you begin this experiment.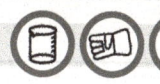

Digestion starts in the mouth. As teeth grind the food, an enzyme in saliva begins the digestion of starch. Other enzymes repeat the process throughout the digestive process. In this experiment, you'll see how starch in food reacts with the salivary enzyme.

Equipment and Materials

5 test tubes	massing paper	dropper	water bath
test tube rack	100-mL graduated cylinder	tincture of iodine	thermometer
balance	1 g potato starch		

Procedure

1. Label five test tubes A through E.
2. In test tube A, place 1 g of potato starch. Add 15 mL of water. Gently flick the test tube to mix.
3. With a dropper, remove a sample of the water-starch mixture from test tube A. Place 20 drops of mixture in test tube B. Add 2 drops of tincture of iodine. Flick tube gently to mix.
4. Record the color of the mixture in each test tube in your data table.
5. Heat a water bath until the thermometer registers 37°C.
6. While the water bath is heating, add approximately 1 cm of saliva to test tube A. Flick the tube to mix. Then place in the water bath.
7. When test tube A has been in the water bath for 5 minutes, remove a sample of the starch-saliva mixture with a dropper. Place 10 drops of the mixture in test tube C. Add 1 drop of tincture of iodine. Gently flick the tube to mix. Then record the color of the mixture in your data table.
8. When test tube A has been in the water bath for 10 minutes, remove another sample of the starch-saliva with a dropper. Place 10 drops in test tube D. Add 1 drop of tincture of iodine and flick tube to mix. Record the color of the mixture in your data table.
9. When test tube A has been in the water bath for 15 minutes, remove a final sample of the starch-saliva mixture with a dropper. Place 10 drops in test tube E. Add 1 drop of tincture of iodine and flick the test tube to mix. Record the color of the mixture in your data table.

(Continued on next page)

EXPERIMENT 13-1 (Continued)

Analyzing Results

1. What color is the mixture when starch is present?

   _____
   _____

2. Was starch present in all the samples tested? If not, when did it disappear?

   _____
   _____
   _____

3. How do you think heat affects enzyme action? How is heat a factor in digestion?

   _____
   _____
   _____
   _____

DATA TABLE

Mixture	Color
Test tube A: starch-water	
Test tube B: water-starch-iodine	
Test tube C: starch-saliva (5 min.)	
Test tube D: starch-saliva (10 min.)	
Test tube E: starch-saliva (15 min.)	

Name _____ Date _____ Class _____

Osmosis

EXPERIMENT 13-2

SAFETY FIRST
Review these safety guidelines before you begin this experiment.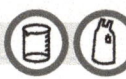

Osmosis is the passage of water and other liquids through a semipermeable membrane. In metabolism, osmosis regulates the concentration of substances on both sides of the membrane.

Eggs contain a membrane through which osmosis can take place. In this experiment, you will determine whether water flows primarily in or out of an egg by observing changes in liquid level and in the size of the egg.

Equipment and Materials

small egg
250-mL beaker
vinegar for soaking egg

water (variation 1)
vinegar (variation 2)
corn syrup (variation 3)

salt (variation 4)
metric ruler
masking tape

marking pen
plastic wrap

Procedure

1. Place an egg in a 250-mL beaker. Add enough vinegar to cover the egg. Let stand for three days to dissolve the shell.
2. Pour out vinegar and carefully rinse any remaining shell off egg, leaving the egg sac.
3. Carefully transfer the egg, which now has no shell, to a clean 250-mL beaker. Follow the variation assigned by your teacher.
   Variation 1. Add water to completely cover the egg.
   Variation 2. Add vinegar to completely cover the egg.
   Variation 3. Add corn syrup to completely cover the egg.
   Variation 4. Add a salt-water solution to completely cover the egg.
4. Measure the height of the liquid in the beaker and record it in your data table.
5. After 30 minutes, again measure the height of the liquid in the beaker. Record in your data table.
6. Label the beaker with your name, variation number, and class. Cover it with plastic wrap. Leave it overnight in the location designated by your teacher.
7. On the following day, measure the liquid height and observe the appearance of the egg and liquid. Note any evidence of layering in the liquid. Record the information in your data table.
8. Record your observations on the heights of your liquid and the appearance of the egg and the liquid on the board. In your data table, copy the results for all variations.

(Continued on next page)

Food Science Lab Manual
Copyright © Mehas & Rodgers

EXPERIMENT 13-2 (Continued)

Analyzing Results

1. In which eggs, if any, did water go into the membrane?

   _____
   _____
   _____

2. In which eggs, if any, did water go out of the membrane?

   _____
   _____
   _____

3. How did you determine whether water went into or out of the membrane?

   _____
   _____
   _____

4. Which eggs lost the most water? Gained the most? Why?

   _____
   _____
   _____
   _____
   _____

(Continued on next page)

Name _____ Date _____ Class _____

EXPERIMENT 13-2 (Continued)

DATA TABLE

Initial Liquid Height	Liquid Height After 30 Minutes	Liquid Height After 24 Hours	Egg Appearance After 24 Hours	Liquid Appearance After 24 Hours
Variation 1: Water				
Variation 2: Vinegar				
Variation 3: Corn Syrup				
Variation 4: Salt-Water				

Kcalories in Food

EXPERIMENT 14-1

SAFETY FIRST
Review these safety guidelines before you begin this experiment.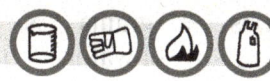

In this chapter, you've seen how food converts to energy during metabolism. Sometimes it's difficult to imagine that a food can actually produce energy. In this experiment, you'll see how burning releases the heat energy in a nut.

Equipment and Materials

shelled nut	coffee can or large juice can	100-mL graduated cylinder
large cork	(top and bottom removed)	laboratory thermometer
long needle	soup can	stirring rod
balance	water	wooden matches

Procedure

1. Create a nut assembly: stick the eye of the needle in the narrow end of the cork, then on the point of the needle mount the shelled nut assigned by your teacher.
2. Determine the mass of the nut assembly. Record it in your data table.
3. Remove both ends of a large can, and punch holes in the sides near the bottom. This will serve as a chimney to minimize heat loss during the experiment.
4. Remove one end of a small aluminum can. Punch two holes, opposite each other, in the sides of the can near the open end.
5. Pour exactly 100 mL of tap water into the small can. Record the temperature of the water in your data table.
6. Insert a glass stirring rod through the holes in the sides of the small can. Use the glass rod to balance the small can within the large can.
7. Place the nut on a nonflammable surface, and ignite it with a match. Immediately place the large can around the nut assembly so the small can of water is above the nut.
8. Allow the nut to burn for 2 minutes or until it goes out.
9. Stir the water with the thermometer. In your data table, record the water's highest temperature.
10. Mass the nut assembly, and record it in your data table.
11. Write your results on the board. Copy the results for the other kinds of nuts in your data table. Expand your data table on separate paper if needed.

(Continued on next page)

EXPERIMENT 14-1 (Continued)

Analyzing Results

1. Using the equation below, calculate the calories of heat from the burning nut. The 100 mL of water has a mass of 100 g.

$$\text{calories} = \text{grams of water} \times \text{degrees of temperature change} \times \text{cal/g°C}$$

_____

_____

2. Divide the figure from question 1 by the change in mass of the nut. This gives the calories released per gram of nut burned. Record this on the board in kcalories.

_____

_____

3. Which kind of nut released the most heat per gram? The least?

_____

_____

_____

4. Do your results agree with the standard calorie tables provided by your teacher? If not, how do you explain any differences between your calculated values for calories per gram and the values listed in the calorie table?

_____

_____

_____

_____

DATA TABLE

Kind of Nut	Mass			Temperature		
	Original	Final	Change	Original	Final	Change

Name _____ Date _____ Class _____

Cellular Respiration

EXPERIMENT 14-2

SAFETY FIRST
Review these safety guidelines before you begin this experiment.

Energy is produced in the cells of the body through the process of cellular respiration. In the lungs, red blood cells absorb oxygen and release carbon dioxide, a waste product of cellular respiration. Respiration rate is measured as the rate at which the body produces carbon dioxide.

In this experiment, you will study the effect of exercise on respiration rate. You will use the indicator bromthymol blue to test for the presence of carbon dioxide in exhaled breath. Bromthymol blue turns yellow in the presence of acid. Since carbon dioxide reacts with water to produce carbonic acid, this indicator can be used to indirectly test for the presence and levels of carbon dioxide in your breath.

Equipment and Materials
2 Erlenmeyer flasks, 250-mL   bromthymol blue solution   2 drinking straws   stopwatch

Procedure
1. Add 150 mL of bromthymol blue solution to each of two Erlenmeyer flasks.
2. Using a straw placed in the solution, exhale into the solution in one of the Erlenmeyer flasks. **Be careful not to inhale any of the solution.**
3. When you begin exhaling into the solution, your partner should start the stopwatch. In your data table, record the time in seconds required for the solution to turn yellow.
4. Now have your partner time you while you do jumping jacks for 30 seconds. If for health reasons you cannot safely exercise at this level, do a less strenuous exercise for a similar time period.
5. Immediately after you stop exercising, use a straw to exhale into the second Erlenmeyer flask. Your partner should again time how long you exhale before the bromthymol blue solution turns yellow. Record this time in your data table.
6. Rinse out the two Erlenmeyer flasks. Add new 150-mL portions of bromthymol blue solution to each one.
7. Repeat Steps 2-5, reversing roles with your partner. You and your partner should do the same exercise, whether jumping jacks or another form.

(Continued on next page)

EXPERIMENT 14-2 (Continued)

Analyzing Results

1. How did the time needed for the bromthymol blue solution to turn yellow before you exercised compare to the time needed after exercising?

   _____

   _____

2. What does the difference in times tell you about your respiration rate in these two situations? How did you reach this conclusion?

   _____

   _____

   _____

   _____

3. Compare your time with your partner's time for each trial of the experiment. What might explain any difference in respiration rates between you and your partner?

   _____

   _____

   _____

   _____

DATA TABLE

Condition	Time for Color Change: Self	Time for Color Change: Partner
Resting		
After exercise		

Name _____ Date _____ Class _____

Thickening Agents

EXPERIMENT 15-1

SAFETY FIRST
Review these safety guidelines before you begin this experiment.

Viscosity is a desirable physical property in many foods. To obtain the desired viscosity in a given recipe, a variety of starches could be used as ingredients. Each of these behaves differently. In this experiment, you'll compare how thickening agents used in food can affect the final product.

Equipment and Materials

starch sample
balance
water
100-mL graduated cylinder
400-mL glass beaker
heat-diffusing ring (for electric ranges)
stirring rod
safety goggles
clear pie plate
line-spread test sheet
plastic ring
saucepan
paper muffin tin liners
masking tape
marking pen
muffin tins

Procedure

1. Obtain a starch from your teacher. Record the type of starch in your data table.
2. Mass a 16-g sample of the starch.
3. Place 60 mL of cold water in a 400-mL beaker; stir in the starch sample. Add 220 mL more water; stir again.
4. Heat the beaker over moderate heat. Stir slowly but constantly until the mixture boils. Wear safety goggles throughout the heating process.
5. Place a glass plate over the line-spread test sheet provided by your teacher. Place a plastic ring in the center of the plate; fill the ring with some of the starch mixture. Lift the ring and allow the mixture to flow for 2 minutes. Count the lines covered at each of 4 points around the circle. Average your readings. Record the result in your data table and on the board.
6. Cool the rest of the starch mixture to room temperature by placing the beaker in a pan of cold water.
7. Repeat the line-spread test described in Step 5, using the cooled mixture.
8. Label two paper muffin cups with your name, and the name of the starch used in the sample. Fill each cup with the starch mixture and place in separate muffin tins. Refrigerate one cup and freeze the other until the next class.
9. On the next day, thaw the frozen sample. Check the thawed and refrigerated samples for retrogradation and syneresis. Record your observations in your data table and on the board. In your data table, also record the results from the other starches written on the board.

(Continued on next page)

Food Science Lab Manual
Copyright © Mehas & Rodgers

EXPERIMENT 15-1 (Continued)

Analyzing Results

1. Compare the findings. Then explain which starches, if any, you would choose to:

   a. Make a molded chicken salad.

   _____

   _____

   _____

   b. Thicken a fruit pie that would be refrigerated before serving.

   _____

   _____

   _____

   c. Make a gravy.

   _____

   _____

   _____

   d. Thicken a cream pie that would be frozen and thawed before serving.

   _____

   _____

   _____

2. What may have caused the different results produced by different starches?

   _____

   _____

   _____

   _____

   _____

(Continued on next page)

Name _____ Date _____ Class _____

EXPERIMENT 15-1 (Continued)

DATA TABLE

Name of Starch	Line-Spread Average		Appearance of Refrigerated Sample	Appearance of Frozen Sample
	Hot	Cold		

EXPERIMENT 16-7 (continued)

DATA TABLE

Name of Starch	Line-Spread Average		Appearance of Refrigerated Sample	Appearance of Frozen Sample
	Hot	Cold		

Name _____ Date _____ Class _____

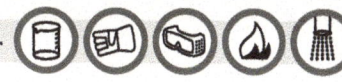

Making Fondant

SAFETY FIRST
Review these safety guidelines before you begin this experiment.

In this experiment, you will discover how temperature, agitation, and the presence of interfering agents affect crystal formation. You will use sugar as a solute and water as a solvent.

Equipment and Materials

sugar
hot water
cream of tartar (variation 2)
corn syrup (variation 3)
half-and-half (variation 5)
balance
saucepan
candy thermometer
100-mL graduated cylinder
safety goggles
heatproof tray
plastic or wooden spoon
plastic wrap
masking tape
marking pen
glycerol
toothpick
microscope
microscope slide

Procedure

1. Based on the control recipe below, follow the recipe variation assigned by your teacher.

Control Recipe for Fondant
200 g sugar
120 mL hot water

Variation 1. Use the control recipe as is.
Variation 2. Use the control recipe, adding 0.3 g of cream of tartar.
Variation 3. Use the control recipe, adding 12 g of corn syrup.
Variation 4. Use the control recipe but do not cool the solution as instructed in Step 6. Beat the mixture until it is white and dry. Then follow the remaining steps.
Variation 5. Use the control recipe but use half-and-half instead of water.

2. Measure the ingredients for the variation you are to make.
3. Place the ingredients in a small saucepan over medium heat. Cover the container and heat until just boiling. This will take about 2 minutes. Wear safety goggles during heating.
4. Remove the cover and boil until the temperature reaches 114°C. Be sure the thermometer has been calibrated.
5. Remove from heat and pour onto a heatproof tray or plate. Use caution when pouring the hot solution.
6. Cool undisturbed until the bottom of the tray or plate is just warm to the touch.
7. Beat vigorously and continuously with a plastic or wooden spoon until the mixture becomes a creamy white mass.
8. Fold, press, and squeeze the mixture until smooth and elastic. Wrap the fondant in plastic film; label with your name, variation, and class. Place the wrapped sample in the location specified by your teacher.
9. The next day, mix a small amount of the sample with a drop of glycerol on a microscope slide, using a toothpick. Examine the sample under a microscope at 10X power.
10. Look through each other's microscopes to view different variations.

(Continued on next page)

Food Science Lab Manual
Copyright © Mehas & Rodgers

EXPERIMENT 15-2 (Continued)

11. On separate paper, sketch the crystals from the five variations.

12. Taste a small sample of each variation. Compare the samples on feel, texture, and moistness. Enter the information in your data table.

Analyzing Results

1. Which variation produced the smallest crystals? The largest crystals? What explains these results?

   _____
   _____
   _____
   _____
   _____
   _____

2. How did the solution's boiling point compare with that of pure water? What happened to the boiling point as time passed?

   _____
   _____
   _____
   _____
   _____

3. If similar procedures were used in fudge making, which variation(s) would produce the best fudge? Why?

   _____
   _____
   _____
   _____
   _____
   _____

(Continued on next page)

Food Science Lab Manual
Copyright © Mehas & Rodgers

Name _____ Date _____ Class _____

EXPERIMENT 15-2 (Continued)

DATA TABLE

Variation	Feel of Crystals on Tongue	Texture	Moistness
1			
2			
3			
4			
5			

Name _____ Date _____ Class _____

EXPERIMENT 15-2 (Continued)

DATA TABLE

Variation	Feel of Crystals on Tongue	Texture	Moistness
1			
2			
3			
4			
5			

Food Science Lab Manual
Copyright © Mebas & Rodgers

133

Name _____ Date _____ Class _____

Effect of Light on Flavor

EXPERIMENT 16-1

SAFETY FIRST
Review these safety guidelines before you begin this experiment.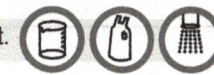

To choose an appropriate packaging method for a food requires knowing the properties of the food, the microorganisms (if any) that affect the food, and how the food changes as its quality deteriorates. As you know, over time, fat oxidizes to become rancid, causing undesirable flavors and odors. These flavors sometimes develop in high-fat foods, such as peanut butter, potato chips, and crackers. How these foods are packaged can affect whether they become rancid, since both light and oxygen accelerate oxidation and rancidity.

In this experiment, you will study the effect of light on the flavor of potato chips stored in different environments for a specified period of time.

Equipment and Materials
2 beakers, 400-mL   balance   plastic wrap   marking pen
aluminum foil   30 g of potato chips   masking tape

Procedure

1. Wrap the outside of one beaker completely in aluminum foil. Leave the other unwrapped.
2. Mass the potato chips. Place 15 g in each beaker.
3. Close the foil-wrapped beaker with additional foil to seal it completely.
4. Tightly seal the unwrapped beaker with plastic wrap.
5. Label the beakers with your name and class. Place them in a location specified by your teacher.
6. Sample the potato chips every other day over a period of two weeks. Rate their flavor, using the following scale:

1—Strongly dislike flavor
2—Slightly dislike flavor
3—Neither like nor dislike flavor
4—Like flavor
5—Greatly enjoy flavor

7. Using graph paper, chart your ratings over the course of the experiment on a graph. Let the y-axis (the side) represent the flavor score; use the x-axis (the bottom) to represent the days.

(Continued on next page)

Food Science Lab Manual
Copyright © Mehas & Rodgers

EXPERIMENT 16-1 (Continued)

Analyzing Results

1. As shown on your graph, when did the flavor of each sample begin to deteriorate? When did the difference become pronounced? What caused this change in flavor?

   _____

   _____

   _____

2. Did either sample stay completely fresh? Why do you think this is so?

   _____

   _____

   _____

3. Based on this experiment, how would you store foods with a high risk of rancidity?

   _____

   _____

DATA TABLE

Day	Rating of Chips Exposed to Light	Rating of Chips Protected from Light	Day	Rating of Chips Exposed to Light	Rating of Chips Protected from Light
1			9		
3			11		
5			13		
7			15		

136   Food Science Lab Manual
Copyright © Mehas & Rodgers

Name _____ Date _____ Class _____

Fat Content of Beef

EXPERIMENT 16-2

SAFETY FIRST
Review these safety guidelines before you begin this experiment.

One way to limit saturated fat in the diet is to buy lean varieties of meat. In this experiment, you will test the fat content of a 100-g sample of ground beef and compare your results with the "percent lean" indicated on the label.

Equipment and Materials

ground beef	600-mL beaker	safety goggles
weighing paper	100-mL graduated cylinder	100-mL beaker
balance		

Procedure

1. Mass 100 g of the ground beef sample assigned by your teacher. Record this value in your data table to the nearest .01 g.
2. Place the ground beef in a 600-mL beaker and add 300 mL of water.
3. Put on safety goggles and heat the mixture until the water boils. Continue heating at a boil for 15 minutes. Heat gently to prevent the liquid from spattering out of the beaker.
4. Remove the beaker from the heat and allow the mixture to cool. The meat will sink to the bottom while the fat rises to the top.
5. Meanwhile, mass a 100-mL beaker. When the sample is cool, carefully pour the fat into the beaker. Mass the beaker and fat; then subtract the mass of the beaker. Record the mass of the fat in your data table.
6. Divide the number of fat grams you recovered by the number of grams of uncooked beef with which you began. Multiply by 100 to obtain the percentage of fat in your sample. Record this information in your data table.
7. In your data table, record the price per pound and the percentage of fat as described on the label of each beef sample.
8. In your data table, record results for the samples checked by other lab groups. Then compare data for all types of ground beef.

Analyzing Results

1. What property of fat molecules allowed you to remove fat from the water?

   _____

   _____

2. According to the experiment, which sample of ground beef had the least fat? Which had the most?

   _____

(Continued on next page)

Food Science Lab Manual
Copyright © Mehas & Rodgers

EXPERIMENT 16-2 (Continued)

3. How did the price per pound of the beef samples compare with their fat content?

   _____

   _____

4. Did the average percentages of fat determined by the class agree with the values on the package labels?

   _____

5. How do you explain any difference between the fat percentages determined in this experiment and the label values?

   _____

   _____

DATA TABLE

Sample ID	Mass of Beef	Mass of Fat	Percentage of Fat	Fat Content Per Label	Price Per Pound

138 Food Science Lab Manual
Copyright © Mehas & Rodgers

Name _____ Date _____ Class _____

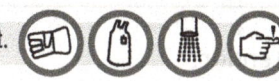
EXPERIMENT 16-3

Lipids and Tenderizing

SAFETY FIRST
Review these safety guidelines before you begin this experiment.

Lipids are an important ingredient in pastries as well as cakes. In this experiment, you will compare the tenderness and mouthfeel of piecrusts prepared with several different lipids.

Equipment and Materials

flour
salt
sifter
hydrogenated shortening (variation 1)
lard (variation 2)
margarine (variation 3)
vegetable oil (variation 4)
balance
mixing bowl
pastry blender (variations 1-3)
100-mL graduated cylinder
fork
rolling pin
cookie sheet
oven mitt or potholder
pizza cutter

Procedure

1. Preheat the oven to 200°C (400°F).
2. Sift together the flour and salt in the control recipe below.

Control Recipe
145 g flour
5 g salt
85 g hydrogenated shortening
water

3. Follow the recipe variation below assigned by your teacher.
   Variation 1. Use the rest of the control recipe as listed. Cut the hydrogenated shortening into the flour-salt mixture.
   Variation 2. Use 85 g of lard instead of hydrogenated shortening. Cut the lard into the flour-salt mixture.
   Variation 3. Use 85 g of margarine instead of hydrogenated shortening. Cut the margarine into the flour-salt mixture.
   Variation 4. Use 85 g of vegetable oil instead of hydrogenated shortening. Stir the vegetable oil into the flour-salt mixture.
4. Slowly sprinkle water on the dough and mix with a fork until the dough is moistened.
5. Gather the dough into a ball. Roll into a 30-cm square on a lightly floured surface. Transfer the dough onto a cookie sheet and prick with the tines of the fork.
6. Place the dough in the oven and bake for 8 to 10 minutes or until light golden brown. Remove from the oven and cool.
7. Using the pizza cutter, cut the dough into 5-cm squares. Set out samples for test tasting as per your teacher's instructions.
8. Taste a sample of each variation and evaluate the texture, tenderness, and flavor. Record your evaluations in your data table.

(Continued on next page)

Food Science Lab Manual
Copyright © Mehas & Rodgers

EXPERIMENT 16-3 (Continued)

Analyzing Results

1. Which crust had the most crisp, flaky texture?

   _____

2. Which crust was the most tender?

   _____

3. Which crust had the best flavor?

   _____

4. How do you explain each of the results you identified in questions 1-3?

   _____
   _____
   _____
   _____

5. Would you expect the lipid that produced the best crust to also produce the best cake? Why or why not?

   _____
   _____
   _____
   _____

DATA TABLE

Variation	Texture	Tenderness	Flavor
1			
2			
3			
4			

140   Food Science Lab Manual
Copyright © Mehas & Rodgers

Name _____ Date _____ Class _____

The Effect of Acid on Protein

EXPERIMENT 17-1

SAFETY FIRST
Review these safety guidelines before you begin this experiment.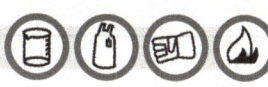

In this experiment you'll compare the behavior of egg white in pure water and in an acid, vinegar, as temperature increases. You will be able to draw some conclusions about the effect of acids on protein in egg white during cooking.

Equipment and Materials
egg white   2 beakers, 100-mL   2 large saucepans
white vinegar   metal spoon   safety goggles
water

Procedure

1. Obtain an egg white sample from your teacher.
2. Pour white vinegar into a 100-mL beaker to a depth of about 3 cm. Pour room-temperature water into a second 100-mL beaker to exactly the same depth as the vinegar.
3. Scoop up 5 mL of egg white. Avoid the chalaza, if possible. Gently add the white to the beaker of water, with a minimum of dripping and stirring. Try to keep the egg white intact. Add 5 mL of egg white to the beaker of vinegar in the same manner.
4. Pour tap water into a large saucepan to a depth of about 3 cm. Heat until the water boils. Wear safety goggles during heating.
5. Pour cold tap water into a second large saucepan to a depth of about 2 cm. Place both 100-mL beakers in this saucepan. Stir the cold water as you slowly add the boiling water. Do not pour any water in the beakers. Stop adding boiling water when the water in the pan is about twice as deep as the liquid in the beakers.
6. Observe the egg samples after they have warmed for 1 minute and again after 3 minutes. Record your observations in your data table.
7. After 5 minutes, remove both beakers from the water bath. Hold them up to examine the samples from the side. Record your observations in your data table.

(Continued on next page)

Food Science Lab Manual
Copyright © Mehas & Rodgers

EXPERIMENT 17-1 (Continued)

Analyzing Results

1. What differences did you observe between the egg white cooked in water and the egg white cooked in vinegar? What caused these differences?

___

2. What substances might you substitute for vinegar to get a similar effect?

___

3. How might you apply your findings when preparing food?

___

DATA TABLE

Time	Egg White in Water	Egg White in Vinegar
1 minute		
3 minutes		
5 minutes		

Name _____ Date _____ Class _____

Egg Foam Stability

EXPERIMENT 17-2

SAFETY FIRST
Review these safety guidelines before you begin this experiment.

An egg foam is formed by beating egg white. Denatured by beating, the egg protein forms a colloidal dispersion, with the air trapped in the white. Several factors affect the stability of a foam. In this experiment, you will add sugar at different points in the beating process and observe its effects on foam formation.

During the beating process, you will need to recognize certain stages in the development of the foam. The *foamy stage* is bubbly and without body. When the *soft peaks stage* is reached, you'll see mounds that look shiny and moist and bend somewhat at the tips when you withdraw the beater. At the *stiff peaks stage*, the mounds elongate and the tips don't bend; the foam will not slip when the bowl is tipped.

Equipment and Materials

sugar
balance
egg
small glass mixing bowl

150-mL beaker
electric or hand mixer
clock or watch with second hand

metric ruler
100-mL graduated cylinder
funnel

Procedure

1. Mass 25 g of sugar.
2. Carefully separate one egg white from its yolk; put the white in a small, glass mixing bowl. Make sure that no yolk gets into the white and that the bowl is clean and grease-free.
3. Follow the variation below assigned by your teacher. When beating the egg white, use a slow or medium speed, as directed by your teacher. When adding sugar, sprinkle it over the egg white.
   Variation 1. Beat the egg white without adding any sugar. Time and record in your data table how long it takes to reach the stiff peaks stage.
   Variation 2. Add all the sugar to the egg white and then begin beating. Time and record in your data table how long it takes to reach the stiff peaks stage.
   Variation 3. Start timing as you beat the egg white. At the foamy stage, begin to add sugar gradually while you continue beating. Add about 5 g of sugar at a time. Continue to time how long it takes for stiff peaks to form. Record the total beating time in your data table.
   Variation 4. Start timing as you beat the egg white. At the soft peaks stage, begin to add sugar gradually while you continue beating. Add about 5 g of sugar at a time. Continue to time how long it takes for stiff peaks to form. Record the total beating time in your data table.
4. Measure the average height of the resulting foam in your variation. Do this by immersing a plastic metric ruler midway between the highest and lowest points in the foam. Record the height in your data table.
5. Using a 100-mL graduated cylinder, measure 75 mL of foam. Place the foam in a funnel supported in a graduated cylinder. Cover and let stand for 20 minutes. In your data table, record the volume of the leakage.
6. Record your data on the board. In your data table, copy the data from the other variations.

(Continued on next page)

Food Science Lab Manual
Copyright © Mehas & Rodgers

EXPERIMENT 17-2 (Continued)

Analyzing Results

1. Which sample gave the greatest height (largest volume) of foam?

   _____

2. Which sample was beaten for the longest time? Did this variation also attain the greatest volume?

   _____

3. Which sample had the greatest volume of leakage?

   _____

4. If sugar is used in a recipe that calls for making a foam from egg whites, when is the best time to add the sugar? Why do you think this is so?

   _____

   _____

DATA TABLE

Variation	Total Beating Time	Height in cm	Leakage in mL
1. No sugar added			
2. All sugar added first			
3. Sugar added gradually from foamy stage			
4. Sugar added gradually from soft peaks stage			

144   Food Science Lab Manual
Copyright © Mehas & Rodgers

Name _____ Date _____ Class _____

Iron as an Additive in Cereals

EXPERIMENT 18-1

SAFETY FIRST
Review these safety guidelines before you begin this experiment.

Many cereals sold in the United States today have iron added to them. This is intended to help consumers meet the minimum daily value recommended for this important mineral. In this experiment you'll compare the amounts of iron present in servings of different cereals.

Equipment and Materials

plastic bag	magnetic stirrer	400-mL beaker	crucible tongs or forceps
cereal sample	magnetic stirring bar	250-mL beaker	paper towel

Procedure

1. In the plastic bag, crush enough of the cereal assigned to you by your teacher to produce a 150-mL sample.
2. Carefully examine the magnetic stirring bar. Describe its appearance in your data table.
3. Place the magnetic stirring bar in a 400-mL beaker. Carefully pour the crushed cereal into the beaker; avoid spilling any. Add 250 mL of water.
4. Place the beaker on a magnetic stirrer and stir for 15 minutes.
5. Using crucible tongs or forceps, remove the stirring bar from the mixture and put it on a paper towel to dry.
6. Observe the appearance of the stirring bar and again record your observations in your data table. Add results of others in the class to your data table. Expand your table on separate paper if necessary.

Analyzing Results

1. Did all of the cereals tested produce a coating of iron on the magnetic stirring bar? Explain.

   _____
   _____

2. Which brand of cereal appeared to have the largest quantity of iron in a 150-mL sample?

   _____

3. How much iron does someone your age and gender need on a daily basis?

   _____
   _____

(Continued on next page)

Food Science Lab Manual
Copyright © Mehas & Rodgers

EXPERIMENT 18-1 (Continued)

4. Based on the information in the Nutrition Facts panel on the cereal box, would a bowl of any of these cereals meet your daily requirement? Explain.

_____

_____

_____

_____

_____

DATA TABLE

Brand of Cereal	Appearance of Bar Before Stirring	Appearance of Bar After Stirring

Name _____ Date _____ Class _____

EXPERIMENT 18-2
Titration of Vitamin C

SAFETY FIRST
Review these safety guidelines before you begin this experiment.

Certain factors cause vitamin C to break down into other compounds. In this experiment, you will test the effect of heat on vitamin C content in apple and orange juice. You will use titration, a way to find the concentration of one substance by using a known amount and concentration of another substance.

This experiment uses an oxidizing agent as an indicator. The amount of the 2,6 dichloroindophenol needed to oxidize the juice sample is proportional to the amount of acid in the juice.

Equipment and Materials
safety goggles
250-mL beaker
orange juice or apple juice
deionized water
100-mL graduated cylinder
50-mL buret
ring stand and clamp
250-mL Erlenmeyer flask
oxalic acid solution
2,6 dichloroindophenol solution

Procedure

1. Wear safety goggles throughout this experiment.
2. If you have been assigned variation 1 or 2, obtain 50 mL of orange juice. If you have been assigned variation 3 or 4, obtain 50 mL of apple juice.
3. Follow the variation assigned.
   Variation 1. Add 50 mL of deionized water to the refrigerated orange juice sample.
   Variation 2. Heat the orange juice sample for 5 minutes on medium heat (1½ minutes in a microwave oven). After heating, add 50 mL deionized water to the sample.
   Variation 3. Use the refrigerated apple juice as is.
   Variation 4. Heat the apple juice sample for 5 minutes on medium heat (1½ minutes in a microwave oven).
4. Clamp a clean 50-mL buret to a ring stand. Fill the buret with the 2,6 dichloroindophenol solution. Read this initial volume and record it in your first data table. Recall that accurate measurements are very important in titration.
5. Place 10 mL of juice into a 250-mL Erlenmeyer flask and add 15 mL of oxalic acid solution.
6. Place the Erlenmeyer flask under the tip of the buret. Release the 2,6 dichloroindophenol solution (a blue oxidizing agent), into the juice solution, drop by drop. When a pink color appears, gently swirl the flask until the color disappears. Swirl after each drop, until 1 drop turns the solution a pink color that does not disappear when the flask is swirled. In your first data table, record the final volume reading from the buret.
7. Repeat the titration two more times, for a total of three titrations. In your data table, record your initial and final buret readings for each titration.
8. To find the volume of base used in each titration, subtract the difference between the initial and final volumes. Record these in your first data table.
9. Average the volumes used in the three trials and record this in your first data table. Write this average on the board.

(Continued on next page)

Food Science Lab Manual
Copyright © Mehas & Rodgers

EXPERIMENT 18-2 (Continued)

10. If more than one lab group in the class tested a variation, average the volumes used for that variation. Record the average volume used for each variation in your second data table.
11. Calculate the milligrams of vitamin C in 100 mL of juice (a typical serving) for each variation, using the equation below. Your teacher will tell you what number to use as the "difference in buret readings for a standard solution."

$$\text{mg vitamin C in 100 mL juice} = \frac{10 \times \text{difference in buret readings}}{\text{difference in buret readings for a standard solution}}$$

Enter this information in your data table.

Analyzing Results

1. Which variation averaged the highest in vitamin C? The lowest?

___

2. How did heat affect the vitamin C content of the juices? Which juice was affected more, orange or apple?

___

3. What storage procedures would you recommend to maintain high levels of vitamin C in apple and orange juice?

___

(Continued on next page)

148   Food Science Lab Manual
Copyright © Mehas & Rodgers

Name _____ Date _____ Class _____

EXPERIMENT 18-2 (Continued)

DATA TABLE
Variation _____

Trial	Individual Buret Readings		
	Initial Volume	Final Volume	Difference (Volume Used)
1			
2			
3			
	Average Volume Used in Variation		

Class Averages

Variation	Average Volume Used in Variations	Average Mg Vitamin C Per 100 mL Juice
1		
2		
3		
4		

Food Science Lab Manual
Copyright © Mehas & Rodgers

EXPERIMENT 18-2 (continued)

DATA TABLE
Variation _____

Trial	Initial Volume	Final Volume	Difference (Volume Used)
1			
2			
3			
Average Volume Used in Variation			

Class Averages

Variation	Average Volume Used in Variations	Average Mg Vitamin C Per 100 mL Juice
1		
2		
3		
4		

DATA TABLE

Name _____ Date _____ Class _____

Enzymes in Foods

EXPERIMENT 19-1

SAFETY FIRST
Review these safety guidelines before you begin this experiment.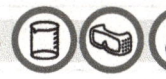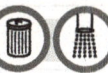

When hydrogen peroxide decomposes, water and oxygen gas form. Catalase is an enzyme that catalyzes the decomposition of hydrogen peroxide to form these products. Only if catalase is present will the oxygen gas result. In this experiment, you will observe the production of oxygen gas when catalase is present. This is the same reaction you've seen if you've ever put hydrogen peroxide on a cut or open wound. In those situations catalase in your blood reacted with the hydrogen peroxide.

Equipment and Materials

hydrogen peroxide   6 beakers, 100-mL   burner or hotplate
food samples   10-mL graduated cylinder

Procedure

1. Obtain two samples each of three different foods, as directed by your teacher; place each sample in a 100-mL beaker, covering the bottom.
2. To only one beaker of each food, add enough water to cover the sample. Place the beakers with water on a burner and heat until the water boils. Continue heating until each food sample is tender.
3. Remove the cooked samples from the burner and carefully drain off the water.
4. Label the beakers, or set them on paper marked with the contents of the beaker. Use your 10-mL graduated cylinder to add 10 mL of hydrogen peroxide to each of the six beakers containing the food samples.
5. In each case record in your data table whether or not bubbling occurred, and if so, to what extent.
6. Dispose of materials as directed by your teacher.

Analyzing Results

1. Which raw sample produced the greatest degree of bubbling?

_____

2. Which cooked sample bubbled the most?

_____

(Continued on next page)

EXPERIMENT 19-1 (Continued)

3. Based on your observations, what effect does cooking have on enzymes?

_____

_____

_____

DATA TABLE

Food Sample	Observations: Cooked	Observations: Uncooked

Name _____ Date _____ Class _____

Enzymatic Browning

EXPERIMENT 19-2

SAFETY FIRST
Review these safety guidelines before you begin this experiment.

Fruit leather is a snack that is easily made with either fresh or canned fruit. Light-colored fruit leather, such as apple or pear, tends to darken during drying because of enzymatic browning. In this experiment, you will test three substances and heat for effectiveness in the creation of fruit leather. **Note:** Because some people have an allergic reaction to bisulfite, *you will not eat the fruit leather containing the bisulfite.*

Equipment and Materials

fruit	10-mL graduated cylinder	rubber spatula
paring knife	ascorbic acid tablets (variations 1, 2)	plastic wrap
cutting board	sodium bisulfite (variations 3, 4)	masking tape
medium saucepan	lemon juice (variations 5, 6)	marking pen
balance	blender or food processor	food dehydrator

Procedure

1. Wash the fruit provided by your teacher.
2. Peel and core the fruit, using a cutting board. Cut away blemishes.
3. Cut the fruit into cubes about 1 cm per side.
4. Follow the variation assigned by your teacher.
   Variation 1. Cook the pieces of fruit in a saucepan over medium heat for 15 minutes, stirring constantly. (A higher temperature may cause the fruit to scorch.) Remove from heat; cool at room temperature for 5 minutes. Crush 375 mg ascorbic acid tablets. Add to the fruit.
   Variation 2. Crush 375 mg ascorbic acid tablets. Add to the cubed fruit.
   Variation 3. Cook the fruit as described in variation 1. Add 0.5 g sodium bisulfite to the fruit.
   Variation 4. Add 0.5 g sodium bisulfite to the cubed fruit.
   Variation 5. Cook the fruit as described in variation 1. Measure 2 mL of lemon juice in the 10-mL graduated cylinder and add to the fruit.
   Variation 6. Measure 2 mL of lemon juice in the 10-mL graduated cylinder and add to the cubed fruit.
5. Purée the fruit in a blender or food processor until it has the thickness of applesauce.
6. Pour the purée onto plastic wrap and spread to 0.5 cm thickness. Label the plastic wrap with your name, class, and variation number.
7. Dry in a dehydrator, maintaining a temperature of 117°-122°C (135°-140°F). (The low drying temperatures will not melt the plastic wrap.) Drying time will vary from 4 to 8 hours. When done, the leather will feel tacky but contain no juice.
8. Cut the fruit leathers made with ascorbic acid and lemon juice for taste testing as directed by your teacher.
9. Evaluate all fruit leathers for color. Describe the flavor and texture of those made with ascorbic acid and lemon juice. Do not taste the fruit leathers made in variations 3 and 4. Enter your observations in your data table.

(Continued on next page)

EXPERIMENT 19-2 (Continued)

Analyzing Results

1. In which fruit leather did the most enzyme activity occur? The least? What evidence supports these conclusions?

   _____

   _____

2. Was color preserved better in the cooked or the uncooked fruit? What explains this result?

   _____

   _____

3. Which of the three additives most effectively preserved the fruit color?

   _____

4. Of the samples tasted, which had the best flavor?

   _____

5. What difference in texture, if any, did you note among the samples?

   _____

   _____

6. Of the methods tested, which produced the overall best fruit leather?

   _____

DATA TABLE

Variation	Color	Flavor	Texture
1			
2			
3		Do not taste.	
4		Do not taste.	
5			
6			

154 Food Science Lab Manual

Name _____ Date _____ Class _____

Effect of Blanching on Enzymes

EXPERIMENT 19-3

SAFETY FIRST
Review these safety guidelines before you begin this experiment.

Freezing is a relatively simple method of preserving food. Although freezing slows down enzyme activity, it does not stop it. Unless frozen food is pretreated, enzyme activity will continue. Blanching is a way to deactivate enzymes with heat. In this experiment, you will observe the effects of blanching on the quality of frozen vegetables.

Equipment and Materials
- fresh vegetables
- paring knife
- peeler (optional)
- 2 saucepans
- safety goggles
- slotted spoon
- bowl and ice water
- paper towels
- 2 plastic freezer bags
- masking tape
- marking pen
- salt

Procedure

1. Prepare the sample of vegetables as instructed by your teacher.
2. Rinse the vegetables thoroughly in cold water. Divide the vegetables into two samples.
3. Fill a large saucepan with water and heat to a rolling boil. Wear safety goggles during heating.
4. Blanch half the vegetables by putting them in the boiling water for 3 minutes. Immediately place the vegetables in ice water. Cool the vegetables in the ice water for 5 minutes; then dry them.
5. Dry the other half of the vegetables without blanching.
6. Pack the vegetables in small plastic freezer bags. Label the bags with your name and class, and indicate whether the vegetables are blanched or unblanched.
7. Freeze the vegetables at −18°C; keep frozen for 3 weeks or longer.
8. After the holding period, add water to two saucepans to a depth of 1 cm. Bring the water in both pans to a boil, and add a pinch of salt to each. Add the package of blanched frozen vegetables to one saucepan and the unblanched vegetables to the other. Reduce heat to low, cover, and cook until the vegetables are done.
9. Evaluate the vegetables for color, aroma, taste, and texture. In your data table, describe these qualities.

(Continued on next page)

EXPERIMENT 19-3 (Continued)

Analyzing Results

1. Why were the vegetables cooled after blanching?

   _____

   _____

2. Which treatment yielded vegetables with better overall quality? How do you explain this result?

   _____

   _____

   _____

   _____

3. How might the results have been different if you had frozen the vegetables only a few days before cooking? Explain your reasoning.

   _____

   _____

   _____

   _____

DATA TABLE

Treatment	Color	Aroma	Taste	Texture
Blanched				
Unblanched				

Name _____ Date _____ Class _____

Temperature and Solubility

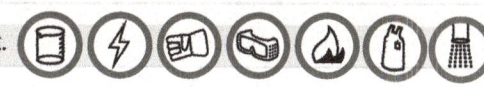

EXPERIMENT 20-1

SAFETY FIRST
Review these safety guidelines before you begin this experiment.

When molecules or ions are pulled apart by the molecules of a solvent, the solvent is said to have dissolved the solute. While the rate at which a solute dissolves is always increased by raising the temperature, the amount of a substance that ultimately dissolves—the solubility of the substance—varies from one solute to another. In this experiment you'll compare the effect of temperature on the solubility of two solids, sodium chloride and sucrose, as well as on carbon dioxide gas.

Equipment and Materials
sodium chloride
sucrose
club soda
water
balance

3 test tubes
2, #2 rubber stoppers, optional
10-mL graduated cylinder
metric ruler

400-mL beaker
burner or hotplate
safety goggles
thermometer

Procedure

1. Mass a 10-g sample of sodium chloride and pour it into a clean test tube.
2. Mass a 10-g sample of sucrose and pour it into another clean test tube.
3. Using your 10-mL graduated cylinder, add 10 mL of room-temperature water (approximately 20°C) to each test tube. Stopper the test tubes or cover with your thumb and shake each tube for 2 minutes to dissolve as much solid as possible.
4. Allow the undissolved solid to settle to the bottom of the test tubes until the liquid above the solid is clear. Measure the height of the remaining solid. Record this information in your data table.
5. Fill a 400-mL beaker half full of water. Place both test tubes in the beaker. Remove stoppers, if used. Place a thermometer in the water in the beaker.
6. Measure 10 mL of club soda, using your 10-mL graduated cylinder, and add it to a third clean test tube. Record the rate of bubbling in your data table. Place this test tube in the 400-mL beaker with the other test tubes.
7. After putting on safety goggles, heat the beaker on a burner set on high until the water temperature reaches 80°C. Note any changes in appearance as the test tubes and their contents are heated.
8. Remove the test tubes from the beaker and place them in a test tube rack. Use your ruler to measure the height of the solid remaining in any of the tubes.

(Continued on next page)

Food Science Lab Manual
Copyright © Mehas & Rodgers

157

EXPERIMENT 20-1 (Continued)

Analyzing Results

1. Describe any difference in the behavior of the solutes as the solutions were heated.

___

2. Which substance(s) seemed to increase in solubility as the temperature rose? Which substance(s) decreased in solubility? Did the solubility of any of the solutes seem to remain the same as the temperature increased?

___

3. Why is it easier to dissolve sugar in hot tea than in iced tea?

___

4. Why is it best to store open containers of carbonated beverages in the refrigerator?

___

(Continued on next page)

Name _____ Date _____ Class _____

EXPERIMENT 20-1 (Continued)

DATA TABLE

Substance	Height of Solid in 20°C Water	Height of Solid in 80°C Water	Observations
Sodium chloride			
Sucrose			

DATA TABLE

	First Rate of Bubbling	Rate of Bubbling After Heating	Observations in 80°C Water
Club soda (containing carbon dioxide)			

Food Science Lab Manual
Copyright © Mehas & Rodgers

Name _____ Date _____ Class _____

Making an Emulsion

EXPERIMENT 20-2

SAFETY FIRST
Review these safety guidelines before you begin this experiment.

Mayonnaise is an emulsion of oil in water. This experiment is designed to illustrate one of the factors that influence the formation of emulsions.

Equipment and Materials
- egg yolks
- balance
- salt (sodium chloride)
- dry mustard
- vinegar
- mixing bowl
- salad oil
- 100-mL graduated cylinder
- 250-mL beaker
- electric mixer

Procedure

1. Measure the ingredients for the control recipe for mayonnaise. Follow the recipe variation in Step 2 as assigned by your teacher.

Control Recipe for Mayonnaise
- 2 egg yolks
- 4.2 g salt
- 1 g dry mustard
- 45 mL vinegar
- 250 mL salad oil

2. Place egg yolks, salt, dry mustard, and 5 mL of vinegar in a small bowl. Beat with an electric mixer at medium speed until the egg yolks are sticky and lemon-colored.

Variation 1. Add the oil drop by drop, beating constantly, until you have added 125 mL of oil. Beat constantly as you slowly add the remaining oil in a thin stream.

Variation 2. Add the oil 5 mL at a time, beating constantly, until you have added 125 mL of oil. Beat constantly as you slowly add the remaining oil in a thin stream.

Variation 3. Add the oil 15 mL at a time, beating constantly until you have added 125 mL oil. Beat constantly as you slowly add the remaining oil in a thin stream.

Variation 4. Add the oil 125 mL at a time, beating constantly until all the oil has been added.

3. Slowly beat the mixture as you add the remaining vinegar in a slow, steady stream.
4. Inspect and sample all four variations of the mayonnaise. Record your observations in your data table.

(Continued on next page)

Food Science Lab Manual
Copyright © Mehas & Rodgers

EXPERIMENT 20-2 (Continued)

Analyzing Results

1. What, if any, were the most significant differences among the variations?

   _____

   _____

   _____

   _____

2. Which variation was the most similar to the mayonnaise found in supermarkets?

   _____

3. What effect did the rate of adding oil have on the quality of the mayonnaise?

   _____

   _____

4. How do you explain the conclusion you reached for question 3?

   _____

   _____

   _____

DATA TABLE

Variation	General Appearance	Color	Flavor	Texture
1				
2				
3				
4				

162   Food Science Lab Manual
Copyright © Mehas & Rodgers

Name _____ Date _____ Class _____

Sensory Evaluation of Gelatin Dessert

EXPERIMENT 20-3

SAFETY FIRST
Review these safety guidelines before you begin this experiment.

In this experiment you will use sensory testing to examine and identify the flavors of three gelatin dessert samples.

Equipment and Materials
3 paper cups
marking pen
spoons
three flavors of prepared gelatin dessert, labeled with three-digit numbers
water glass or cup

Procedure
1. Label each paper cup with one of the identification numbers from the containers of gelatin dessert. Spoon a small amount of that sample into the cup.
2. Taste the sample. Record your responses in your data table, including what you believe the flavor to be.
3. Rinse your mouth with water.
4. Taste the remaining two samples in the same manner.
5. After all students have completed their taste tests, your teacher will identify the flavor of each sample.

Analyzing Results

1. Which of your senses did you use most to evaluate the flavor of the samples?

   _____

2. Of the four main tastes (salty, sour, bitter, sweet), which did your taste buds detect most?

   _____

3. Did any flavor taste sweeter than any others? If so, which one? What might explain this?

   _____

   _____

   _____

(Continued on next page)

Food Science Lab Manual
Copyright © Mehas & Rodgers

EXPERIMENT 20-3 (Continued)

4. What created the texture of the gelatin samples? How might texture affect the evaluation of flavor?

___

5. What would happen to the volatile substances if the samples were served at room temperature rather than chilled?

___

6. How many of the samples did you correctly identify?

___

DATA TABLE

Sample No.	Color	Aroma	Mouthfeel	Taste	Flavor

Name _____ Date _____ Class _____

Using Baking Powders to Produce Carbon Dioxide

EXPERIMENT 21-1

SAFETY FIRST
Review these safety guidelines before you begin this experiment.

Baking powder releases carbon dioxide gas. In this experiment, you will identify sources of carbon dioxide and compare the approximate amounts of CO_2 produced by each.

Equipment and Materials

albumin solution
2 graduated cylinders, 50-mL or 100-mL
3 beakers, 250-mL
2 different brands of baking powder
sodium bicarbonate (baking soda)
cream of tartar
balance
massing paper
stirring rod or spoon
shallow saucepan or waterbath
safety goggles
masking tape
marking pen
pH indicator paper with 1-11 range
clock for timing
plastic metric ruler

Procedure

1. Place 15 mL of albumin solution in each of three, 250-mL beakers.
2. On squares of paper, mass 3.5 g of two different brands of baking powder.
3. Mass 2 g of sodium bicarbonate and 3.9 g of cream of tartar. Mix them to form baking powder.
4. Place tap water in a shallow container to a depth of about 2.5 cm. Bring water to a simmer. Wear safety goggles during heating.
5. Pour the baking powders into the three, 250-mL beakers at the same time (one powder in each beaker, marked for identification). Stir quickly but only enough to disperse the baking powder. Check pH of foam.
6. At 1-minute intervals for 5 minutes, measure the height of the foam in each beaker. After the final height measurement, determine the liquids' pH with pH paper. Record this information in your data table.
7. After 5 minutes, place the three beakers in the shallow container of simmering water.
8. Heat the beakers for 5 minutes. Measure the height of the foam each minute, and observe changes during that time. Again, test the liquids with pH paper after the final height measurement to determine pH. Record this information in your data table.

Analyzing Results

1. What are the ingredients in baking powder?

_____
_____

(Continued on next page)

Food Science Lab Manual
Copyright © Mehas & Rodgers

165

EXPERIMENT 21-1 (Continued)

2. Which baking powder produced the most foam at room temperature? When heated?
___
___
___

3. Which baking powder was most acidic? Basic?
___
___
___

4. How did heating affect the pH of the solutions?
___
___
___
___
___

DATA TABLE

| Time | Height at Room Temperature | | | pH at Room Temperature | | | Height in Warm Water | | | pH in Warm Water | | |
	Sample #1	#2	#3	Sample #1	#2	#3	Sample #1	#2	#3	Sample #1	#2	#3
1 minute												
2 minutes												
3 minutes												
4 minutes												
5 minutes												

Name _____ Date _____ Class _____

Comparison of Leavening Agents

EXPERIMENT 21-2

SAFETY FIRST
Review these safety guidelines before you begin this experiment.

In this experiment you'll test and compare the effects of various leavening agents.

Equipment and Materials

sugar
cake flour
salt
double-acting baking powder (variations 1, 2, 3)
hydrogenated shortening
milk
vanilla
egg
sodium bicarbonate (variations 4, 5, 6)
cream of tartar (variation 4)

vinegar (variation 5)
buttermilk (variation 6)
balance
100-mL graduated cylinder
10-mL graduated cylinder
150-mL beaker
sifter
mixing bowl
electric mixer
round baking pan
potholders
cooling rack

plastic wrap
masking tape
marking pen
knife
metric ruler
paper towels
deionized water
spoon
small dish or beaker
pH indicator paper

Procedure

1. Use the control recipe below to measure ingredients. Follow the variation assigned to you in order to alter certain measurements. Ingredients should be at room temperature.

Control Recipe for Basic Cake

150 g sugar
108 g cake flour
1.8 g salt
3.5 g double-acting baking powder
47 g hydrogenated shortening
120 mL milk
2 mL vanilla
1 egg (about 41 g)

Variation 1. Use the control recipe as stated.
Variation 2. Increase baking powder to 4.7 g.
Variation 3. Decrease baking powder to 1.7 g.
Variation 4. Replace baking powder with 2 g of sodium bicarbonate plus 3.9 g of cream of tartar.
Variation 5. Replace baking powder with 2 g of sodium bicarbonate. Replace 120 mL of milk with 105 mL of milk plus 15 mL of vinegar. Mix milk with vinegar well.
Variation 6. Replace baking powder with 1 g of sodium bicarbonate. Use buttermilk instead of regular milk.

2. Sift the dry ingredients into a mixing bowl.
3. Add shortening and 80 mL of the liquid to dry ingredients.
4. Beat for 2 minutes at medium speed with an electric mixer or 300 strokes by hand.
5. Add the egg, remainder of the liquid, and vanilla.
6. Beat 2 minutes or 300 strokes more.

(Continued on next page)

Food Science Lab Manual
Copyright © Mehas & Rodgers

EXPERIMENT 21-2 (Continued)

7. Lightly grease and flour a 23-cm (9-in.) round cake pan. Pour in the batter and bake for 20 minutes at 185°C (365°F). Use potholders to remove the pan from the oven.
8. Let the cake cool for 10 minutes; then remove from pan and place on a cooling rack. When cool, wrap in plastic wrap and label with your name, class, and variation. Place in the location specified by your teacher.
9. The next day, slice the cake in half, forming two half circles. Measure the height of the cake at the center, using a metric ruler.
10. Record the height in your data table and on the board. Copy the heights of the other variations in your data table.
11. Cut the remaining cake into small pieces. Put the pieces on a paper labeled with the variation number. Set out for taste testing.
12. Taste samples of each variation; evaluate for texture, tenderness, flavor, and moistness. Record your evaluations in your data table.
13. Mix one piece of each variation with enough deionized water to make a smooth suspension. Use pH paper to determine the pH. Record this information in your data table.

Analyzing Results

1. Which leavening agent produced the tallest cake? The shortest?

_____

_____

2. What effects did the various leavening agents have on texture? Tenderness? Flavor? Moistness?

_____

_____

_____

_____

_____

3. How does the pH of each sample compare with the pH of the leavening used in it? (The pH values of leavening agents were tested in Experiment 21-1.) What would explain any difference between the two levels?

_____

_____

_____

_____

(Continued on next page)

Name _____ Date _____ Class _____

EXPERIMENT 21-2 (Continued)

4. Of the six samples, which did you prefer? Why?

   _____

   _____

   _____

   _____

DATA TABLE

Variation	Height	Texture	Tenderness	Flavor	Moistness	pH
1						
2						
3						
4						
5						
6						

Food Science Lab Manual
Copyright © Mehas & Rodgers

EXPERIMENT 27-2 (Continued)

4. Of the six samples, which did you prefer? Why?

_____

_____

_____

DATA TABLE

Variation	Height	Texture	Tenderness	Flavor	Moistness	pH

Name _____ Date _____ Class _____

Yeast Growth

EXPERIMENT 22-1

SAFETY FIRST
Review these safety guidelines before you begin this experiment.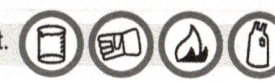

In this experiment, you will grow yeast in a variety of environments to determine how each affects yeast growth.

Equipment and Materials
water
100-mL graduated cylinder
250-mL beaker
saucepan
dry yeast
balance
stirring rod
sucrose
sodium chloride
laboratory thermometer
metric ruler

Procedure
1. Add 100 mL of water to a 250-mL beaker. Heat the water to 35°C over medium heat.
2. Put a small saucepan half full of water on a second burner over low heat.
3. When the temperature of the water in the beaker has reached 35°C, remove it from the heat. Add 3.2 g dry yeast to the beaker and mix thoroughly so all the yeast dissolves.
4. Follow the variation assigned by your teacher.
   Variation 1. Add nothing to the yeast and water mixture.
   Variation 2. Add 4.3 g sugar to the yeast and water; mix well.
   Variation 3. Add 6.6 g of salt to the yeast and water; mix well.
   Variation 4. Add 4.3 g sugar and 6.6 g salt to the yeast and water; mix well.
5. Remove the saucepan from the range. Determine the temperature of the water in the saucepan.
6. Add cool water if necessary to adjust the temperature of the water to 30°C. Place the beaker containing the yeast mixture in the warm water in the saucepan for 15 minutes.
7. After 15 minutes, remove the beaker from the saucepan. Measure the height of the yeast mixture. In your data table, record the height of the mixture for the variation.
8. Observe the odor and consistency of your mixture, and record this information in your data table.
9. Write the information for your variation on the board. In your data table, copy the information for the other variations.

(Continued on next page)

Food Science Lab Manual
Copyright © Mehas & Rodgers

EXPERIMENT 22-1 (Continued)

Analyzing Results

1. In which environment did the yeast grow best? Worst? Why?

   _____
   _____
   _____
   _____

2. Why wasn't the beaker placed directly on the heating element during yeast growth?

   _____
   _____
   _____
   _____

3. Check at least three different bread recipes. Do the ingredients used and directions given agree with the results of this experiment?

   _____
   _____
   _____
   _____
   _____

DATA TABLE

Variation	Height	Odor	Consistency
1			
2			
3			
4			

Name _____ Date _____ Class _____

EXPERIMENT 22-2
Fermentation of Pickles

SAFETY FIRST
Review these safety guidelines before you begin this experiment.

In this experiment, you will prepare pickles from cucumbers. As fermentation proceeds, you will monitor changes in the color and texture of the cucumbers, and in the appearance and pH of the brine.

Equipment and Materials
1000-mL beaker	balance	cucumbers	plastic bag
masking tape	pickling spice	knife	pH indicator paper
marking pen	dill seed	brine	

Procedure
1. Thoroughly wash a 1000-mL beaker. Label with your name and class.
2. Mass 2 g of pickling spice and 2 g of dill seed. Pour the spice and dill seed into the beaker.
3. Wash 4-6 cucumbers, trimming stems if necessary. Place cucumbers in the beaker.
4. Add brine supplied by your teacher until the pickles are completely covered.
5. Fill a plastic bag with brine solution and seal tightly. Place the plastic bag on top of the cucumbers to submerge them in brine.
6. Leave your beaker in the location indicated by your teacher.
7. Every few days, do the following:
   a. Check to see that the cucumbers are covered with brine. Add more if needed.
   b. Skim off any film that forms.
   c. Record the following information in your data table: color of the cucumber/pickles; texture of the cucumbers/pickles; appearance of the brine (clear, cloudy); and pH of the brine as tested with pH paper.
8. Allow the fermentation process to continue for about 5 weeks, or until the pH of the brine stabilizes at 3.5 or below for at least one week. Do not taste the pickles if the pH remains above 4.

Analyzing Results

1. What changes occurred in the color and texture of the cucumbers as they fermented?

_____
_____
_____
_____
_____

(Continued on next page)

Food Science Lab Manual
Copyright © Mehas & Rodgers

EXPERIMENT 22-2 (Continued)

2. What changes occurred in the appearance of the brine?

_____

_____

_____

3. What is the final pH of the brine solution? How does it compare to the pH at the start of fermentation?

_____

_____

4. Is the pH low enough to preserve the pickles? If not, what could you do to lower it?

_____

_____

DATA TABLE

Date	Color	Texture	Appearance of Brine	pH of Brine

Name _____ Date _____ Class _____

Lactic-Acid Fermentation

EXPERIMENT 22-3

SAFETY FIRST
Review these safety guidelines before you begin this experiment.

In this experiment, you will prepare sauerkraut from cabbage. As fermentation proceeds, you will monitor changes in the color and texture of the cabbage, and in the appearance and pH of the brine.

Equipment and Materials

cabbage	balance	masking tape
knife	jar and lid	marking pen
cutting board	wooden spoon	paper towels
mixing bowl	plastic bag	pH indicator paper
sodium chloride	extra brine (if needed)	

Procedure

1. Remove and discard the outer leaves from a firm, mature head of cabbage. Wash, drain, and cut the head in half. (Another lab group will use the other half.) Remove and discard the core.
2. Shred the cabbage, using a sharp knife. Pieces should be no thicker than a dime. Place the shredded cabbage in a mixing bowl.
3. Sprinkle 18.2 g of sodium chloride (salt) over the shredded cabbage, and mix thoroughly by hand. The salt will pull water from the cabbage to form a brine.
4. Pack the cabbage into a clean jar, pressing down firmly with a wooden spoon. Fill the jar to 5 cm from the top. Be sure the brine covers the cabbage. If you need more brine, obtain it from your teacher.
5. Fill a plastic bag with brine provided by your teacher, and seal tightly. Place the plastic bag on top of the cabbage and hold it down. Wipe the top of the jar and place the lid on loosely.
6. Label your jar with your name and class, and place in the location indicated by your teacher.
7. Every few days, do the following:
   a. Check to see that the cabbage is covered with brine. If necessary, add a weak brine made by dissolving 28.8 g salt in 1 L of water.
   b. With a paper towel, skim off any film that forms.
   c. Record the following information in your data table: color of the cabbage/sauerkraut; texture of the cabbage/sauerkraut; appearance of the brine (clear, cloudy); and pH of the brine as tested with pH paper. Expand your data table on separate paper if needed.
8. Allow the fermentation process to continue for about 5 weeks, or until the pH of the brine is 3.5 or below for at least one week. Do not taste the sauerkraut if the pH remains above 4.

(Continued on next page)

Food Science Lab Manual
Copyright © Mehas & Rodgers

EXPERIMENT 22-3 (Continued)

Analyzing Results

1. For what reasons was the cabbage washed before shredding?

   _____
   _____

2. What changes occurred in the color and texture of the cabbage as it fermented?

   _____
   _____
   _____

3. What changes occurred in the appearance of the brine?

   _____
   _____

4. What is the final pH of the brine solution? How does it compare to the pH at the start of fermentation?

   _____
   _____

5. Is the pH low enough to preserve the sauerkraut? If not, what could you do to lower it?

   _____
   _____

DATA TABLE

Date	Color	Texture	Appearance of Brine	pH of Brine

Separating Milk

EXPERIMENT 23-1

SAFETY FIRST
Review these safety guidelines before you begin this experiment.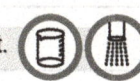

Do you recall the childhood rhyme about Miss Muffet, who ate curds and whey? As you've learned, milk is both a solution and a colloidal dispersion. Normally, the protein molecules in milk, which are too large to dissolve, remain suspended as colloids. Miss Muffet's colloids had clumped into solid curds, which she ate along with the whey, or the remaining liquid. In this experiment you will see what may have produced Miss Muffet's meal.

Equipment and Materials

whole milk	water	100-mL graduated cylinder
vinegar	3, 250-mL beakers	stirring rod
lemon juice		

Procedure

1. Add 100 mL of milk to each of three, clean, dry, 250-mL beakers.
2. After carefully rinsing out your graduated cylinder, measure 30 mL of vinegar and add it to the milk in the first beaker. Stir.
3. Repeat Step 2, adding 30 mL of lemon juice to the second beaker, and then 30 mL of water to the third beaker. Record your observations in your data table.
4. Allow the milk to sit for 1 minute. Record your observations in your data table.
5. Record your observations in your data table after the milk sits for 5 minutes.

Analyzing Results

1. What effect did the vinegar, lemon juice, and water have on the milk?

_____
_____
_____
_____
_____
_____
_____

(Continued on next page)

Food Science Lab Manual
Copyright © Mehas & Rodgers

EXPERIMENT 23-1 (Continued)

2. Why do vinegar and lemon juice affect milk as they do?

   _____
   _____
   _____
   _____

3. What dairy products can you identify that have curds?

   _____
   _____
   _____

DATA TABLE

	Milk with Vinegar	**Milk with Lemon Juice**	**Milk with Water**
Appearance of milk initially			
Appearance of milk after 1 minute			
Appearance of milk after 5 minutes			

178　　Food Science Lab Manual
Copyright © Mehas & Rodgers

EXPERIMENT 23-2
Making Yogurt

SAFETY FIRST
Review these safety guidelines before you begin this experiment.

Yogurt is a cultured milk product made when lactic-acid bacteria cause milk to ferment. The milk is first heated to kill any undesirable bacteria that may be present and to denature the milk protein. This gives the finished product a firmer body and custard-like texture. Lactic-acid bacteria are then inoculated into the milk, and the milk is incubated. This experiment lets you observe the changes caused by lactic-acid bacteria in making yogurt.

Equipment and Materials
- yogurt base
- saucepan or double boiler
- safety goggles
- laboratory thermometer in stopper
- ring stand and clamp
- yogurt maker or a setting pan apparatus
- yogurt culture
- 50-mL beaker
- spoon
- yogurt containers and covers
- pH indicator paper
- ice and pan (optional)

Procedure

1. Obtain a yogurt base (kind of milk) from your instructor. Three different yogurt bases will be used in this experiment.
2. Heat the base assigned to your group in a saucepan or double boiler to 82°C. Maintain this temperature for 15-20 minutes. Wear safety goggles while heating.
3. Cool the yogurt base to 43°C.
4. Add 30 mL of yogurt culture to the 43°C yogurt base. Mix with a gentle stirring motion to minimize the addition of air.
5. Fill yogurt containers and cover. Mark your containers with the code number of your base.
6. Put filled containers in either a yogurt maker or setting pans. Maintain the temperature at 43°C. Check frequently, as temperatures of 46°C and above will kill the culture.
7. When the milk has coagulated and formed a firm gel, remove the yogurt containers. Cool them immediately by setting them in ice or refrigerating.
8. Measure the pH of a sample of each yogurt base and record in your data table.
9. Test a sample of each yogurt base for color, texture, and taste. Record your observations in your data table.

Analyzing Results

1. Were there differences in color among the fermented samples? If so, which looked most appealing?

_____
_____
_____

(Continued on next page)

Food Science Lab Manual
Copyright © Mehas & Rodgers

EXPERIMENT 23-2 (Continued)

2. What textural difference, if any, did you note among the samples?
   _____
   _____

3. Which of the samples, if any, had an unpleasant taste?
   _____
   _____

4. Which sample was the most acidic?
   _____
   _____

5. Is there any correlation between the degree of acidity and taste?
   _____
   _____

6. All factors considered, which base produced the best yogurt?
   _____
   _____

7. Which do you prefer, the best homemade yogurt or the best commercial brand? Why?
   _____
   _____
   _____

DATA TABLE

Yogurt Base No.	pH	Color	Texture	Taste

Name _____ Date _____ Class _____

Evaluation of Commercial Yogurts

EXPERIMENT 23-3

SAFETY FIRST
Review these safety guidelines before you begin this experiment.

Several factors figure prominently in judging the quality of yogurt. Yogurt should have a smooth, uniform texture. No graininess, lumpiness, or liquid whey should be present. Good yogurt has no unpleasant aftertaste. In this experiment, you will evaluate the quality of commercially prepared yogurt.

Note that some yogurt contains live bacteria that have the enzyme lactase, which may aid in lactose digestion. Other yogurt is heat-treated to destroy the bacterial culture. While extending the shelf life, this heat-treatment eliminates any health benefits that might result from the live microorganisms.

Equipment and Materials
yogurt samples   masking tape   spoon
paper plate   marking pen   paper cup

Procedure
1. Attach equally spaced labels around the edge of a paper plate, identifying the numbers of all yogurt samples. Place a bite-size amount of each yogurt sample beside the correct identification number.
2. Evaluate each sample on color, texture, and taste. Using a paper cup, rinse your mouth with water between samples. Record your observations in your data table. Also mark one sample as your favorite.
3. After all students have finished the taste test, your teacher will display the container and the unit price of each sample. In your data table, record the price and the following information from the container:
   a. Brand name
   b. Any colorings and flavorings
   c. Whether the sample contained live bacteria

Analyzing Results
1. Read the list of ingredients for the sample that you judged best in appearance. Which ingredients do you think contributed to this effect?

   _____
   _____

2. Read the list of ingredients for the sample with the best flavor. What ingredients do you think contributed to its taste?

   _____
   _____

(Continued on next page)

Food Science Lab Manual
Copyright © Mehas & Rodgers

3. Read the Nutrition Facts panel of the yogurt you liked best. Is it also a nutritious choice? Explain your answer.

_____
_____
_____

4. Compare the number of kcalories per serving among the different brands. Does the brand you favor provide a reasonable number? Explain.

_____
_____
_____

5. Did the yogurt with the highest unit price seem worth the added cost? If so, in what qualities is it superior?

_____
_____
_____

6. For what reasons would you buy yogurt with or without live bacterial cultures?

_____
_____
_____

DATA TABLE

	Yogurt Samples						
Color							
Texture							
Taste							
Favorite							
Brand							
Unit price							
Colorings							
Flavorings							
Live bacteria?							

Name _____ Date _____ Class _____

Testing for Food Additives

EXPERIMENT 24-1

SAFETY FIRST
Review these safety guidelines before you begin this experiment.

One method of preventing browning in dried fruits is by sulfuring, a technique in which fruits are exposed to sulfur dioxide gas for varying amounts of time. Once the process has been completed, there is no way to tell visually if a fruit has been exposed to the sulfuring process.

In this experiment, you will use a series of chemical reactions to determine whether or not sulfur dioxide was used to preserve the fruit.

Equipment and Materials
dried fruit (two kinds)
400-mL beaker
250-mL beaker
100-mL graduated cylinder
distilled or deionized water
stirring rod
filter paper
funnel
safety goggles
hydrogen peroxide solution
dropper (or dropping bottle)
barium chloride solution

Procedure
1. Place 2–4 pieces of one type of fruit in the 400-mL beaker and cover the fruit with distilled or deionized water.
2. Let the mixture stand for 15 minutes, stirring often with a stirring rod. As the fruit absorbs the water, you may need to add more water to the beaker.
3. Drain the liquid from the fruit through filter paper in a funnel into a clean, dry, 250-mL beaker. This liquid is called the filtrate.
4. After putting on safety goggles, add 50 mL of 3-percent H_2O_2 (hydrogen peroxide) to the filtrate.
5. Using a dropper, add several drops of $BaCl_2$ to the filtrate. If a white solid forms, SO_2 was used to preserve the fruit. If no white solid forms, sulfur dioxide was not used.
6. Repeat the above steps, using another fruit and record all information in your data table. Check with other lab groups to determine the results for fruits you didn't test. Add those results to your table.

Analyzing Results
1. Which of the fruits had been exposed to the sulfuring method of preservation?

_____

_____

(Continued on next page)

Food Science Lab Manual
Copyright © Mehas & Rodgers

2. Why are some fruits exposed to SO₂?

   _____

   _____

   _____

3. What could happen to fruits during shipping or after sitting in a store for long periods of time if SO₂ were not used?

   _____

   _____

   _____

4. What other types of additives may be in the fruits you tested?

   _____

   _____

5. SO₂ is also used to change the color of foods. Raw sugar is brown, but when bleached with SO₂, it becomes white. Why do you think sugar is bleached?

   _____

   _____

   _____

DATA TABLE

Kind of Fruit	White Solid Formed? (yes/no)	Sulfur Dioxide Used? (yes/no)

Pudding Mixes and Additives

EXPERIMENT 24-2

SAFETY FIRST
Review these safety guidelines before you begin this experiment.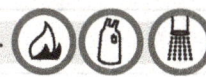

In this experiment, you will observe the effect of additives on vanilla pudding.

Equipment and Materials
vanilla pudding mix	spoon	2 muffin tins
package label from mix	100-mL graduated cylinder	2 paper muffin tin liners
sugar (variation 2)	clear plate	masking tape
lemon juice (variation 3)	line-spread test sheet	marking pen
measuring cup	plastic ring	plastic wrap
small saucepan	large pan of cold water	

Procedure

1. Follow the variation assigned by your teacher.
   Variation 1. Prepare a vanilla pudding mix according to the directions on the package.
   Variation 2. Prepare a vanilla pudding mix, but add 80 g of sugar to the dry mix before adding liquid.
   Variation 3. Prepare a vanilla pudding mix, but substitute lemon juice for the liquid in the recipe. Reduce the amount of lemon juice to one-third the amount of liquid called for.
2. Place a clear plate over the line-spread test sheet provided by your teacher. Place a plastic ring in the center, and fill with the hot cooked pudding. Lift the ring and allow the pudding to flow for 2 minutes. Count the lines covered at each of 4 points around the circle, and average your results. In your data table, record this result for the variation you made.
3. Cool the rest of the pudding to room temperature by placing the saucepan in a pan of cold water.
4. While the pudding cools, list the ingredients on the package label in your lab report. Explain what you believe is the purpose of each ingredient.
5. Repeat the line-spread test described in Step 2 with the room-temperature pudding.
6. Label two paper muffin tin liners with your name, class, and variation number. Place one in each muffin tin. Fill the cups with the pudding mixture, and cover each with plastic wrap. Refrigerate one and freeze the other until the next class begins.
7. Thaw the frozen pudding sample. Examine the thawed and refrigerated samples for retrogradation and syneresis. Record your observations in your data table.
8. Write your data on the board. In your data table, copy the data from the other variations.

(Continued on next page)

EXPERIMENT 24-2 (Continued)

Analyzing Results

1. In what ways were the variations different?

   _____

   _____

   _____

   _____

2. Which variation would you choose if you had to prepare a pudding the night before for a pie filling needed the next day? Why?

   _____

   _____

   _____

   _____

3. Explain the change that occurred when lemon juice was added.

   _____

   _____

   _____

4. What change occurred when sugar was added?

   _____

   _____

   _____

5. What changes occurred when the pudding was refrigerated?

   _____

   _____

   _____

   _____

(Continued on next page)

Food Science Lab Manual
Copyright © Mehas & Rodgers

Name _____ Date _____ Class _____

EXPERIMENT 24-2 (Continued)

6. What changes occurred when the pudding was frozen and thawed?

   _____

   _____

   _____

7. How do you think the additives influenced the behavior of the pudding, as compared with the starches in Experiment 15-1?

   _____

   _____

   _____

   _____

DATA TABLE

Variation	Line-Spread Average		Observations	
	Hot	Room Temp.	Refrigerated Sample	Frozen Sample
1				
2				
3				

Food Science Lab Manual
Copyright © Mehas & Rodgers

Name _____ Date _____ Class _____

Effects of Minerals on Protein

EXPERIMENT 24-3

SAFETY FIRST
Review these safety guidelines before you begin this experiment.

Tofu, a basic part of the diet in Southeast Asia, is a protein product made of soybean curd. It is often used as a meat substitute in the United States. In this experiment, you will compare the effects of the mineral salts, calcium sulfate and magnesium sulfate, on the characteristics of tofu.

Equipment and Materials

dry soybeans	extra-large saucepan	knife
balance	safety goggles	cutting board
1000-mL beaker	cheesecloth	frying pan
masking tape	magnesium sulfate (variation 1)	tablespoon
marking pen	calcium sulfate (variation 2)	margarine
strainer	400-mL beaker	paper plate
blender	400-mL plastic beaker	

Procedure

1. Mass 140 g of dry soybeans. Wash the beans thoroughly, and place them in a 1000-mL beaker containing 500 mL of water. Label the beaker with your name and class. Let the beans soak overnight in the location specified by your teacher.
2. The next day, drain the beans through a strainer and rinse them twice with tap water.
3. Place the rinsed beans in a blender with 250 mL of water, and liquefy.
4. In an extra-large saucepan, bring 1 L of water to a boil. Wear safety goggles while heating.
5. Add the liquefied mixture to the hot water. This mixture is called soymilk.
6. Separate the residue of skins from the soymilk by straining the mixture through six layers of cheesecloth into a kettle.
7. Wearing safety goggles, boil the soymilk over medium-high heat for 3 minutes or until foamy. Remove the kettle from the stove.
8. Follow one variation, as directed by your teacher.
   Variation 1. Slowly stir the mixture as you add 4.5 g of magnesium sulfate.

   Variation 2. Slowly stir the mixture as you add 2.9 g of calcium sulfate.
9. Wait 10 minutes until the soymilk has curdled, forming tofu curds. Place the mixture in fresh cheesecloth in a clean extra-large saucepan. Rinse and squeeze the curds. Allow the curds to drain for 2-3 hours.
10. Mass a clean, dry 400-mL beaker labeled with your name, class, and the variation used. Record the mass in your data table.
11. Put the drained curds into the labeled beaker, cover with cold water, and store overnight in a refrigerator.
12. The next day, drain the curds and mass the beaker and tofu curds. Record the mass in your data table. Calculate the mass of the curds.
13. Write the mass of the curds on the board. In your data table, copy the mass of the curds from other groups for both variations.
14. Cut the tofu into 1-cm cubes.
15. In a frying pan, melt 15 mL of margarine over medium heat. Add one-half the tofu cubes and fry for 5-10 minutes or until light golden brown.

(Continued on next page)

Food Science Lab Manual
Copyright © Mehas & Rodgers

EXPERIMENT 24-3 (Continued)

16. Place the fried and the fresh tofu samples on a paper plate, labeled with the variation used, in the location indicated by your teacher.

17. Sample all variations of tofu. Evaluate for tenderness, texture, and flavor.

Analyzing Results

1. How does the mass of the curds compare with the original mass of beans? Were these results consistent for both variations? What might explain any differences?

_____
_____
_____
_____
_____

2. How do the tofu samples compare in texture? What do you think caused any textural differences?

_____
_____
_____

3. How do you think the samples compare in nutritive value?

_____
_____
_____

4. Which tofu sample do you prefer? Why?

_____
_____
_____
_____

(Continued on next page)

EXPERIMENT 24-3 (Continued)

DATA TABLE

Variation	Mass of Empty Beaker	Mass of Beaker and Curds	Mass of Curds
1			
2			

DATA TABLE

Tofu Sample	Tenderness	Texture	Flavor
Variation 1: *Fresh*			
Variaton 1: *Fried*			
Variation 2: *Fresh*			
Variation 2: *Fried*			

Name _____ Date _____ Class _____

EXPERIMENT 24-3 (Continued)

DATA TABLE

Variation	Mass of Empty Beaker	Mass of Beaker and Curds	Mass of Curds
1			
2			

DATA TABLE

Test Sample	Tenderness	Texture	Flavor
Variation 0, Fresh			
Variation 1, Fresh			
Variation 2, Fresh			
Variation 2, Fresh			

Food Science Lab Manual
Copyright © Mebus & Rodgers

191

Name _____ Date _____ Class _____

Growing Cultures

EXPERIMENT 25-1

SAFETY FIRST
Review these safety guidelines before you begin this experiment.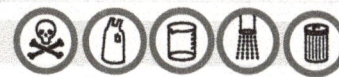

Although single microorganisms are not visible, colonies of microorganisms, called cultures, can be seen. Cultures are grown in the lab on a gelatinous substance called nutrient agar (AH-gar), which promotes bacterial growth. In this experiment, you'll discover just how widespread microorganisms really area.

Equipment and Materials
sterile petri dish filled with agar   cellophane tape   marking pen   masking tape

Procedure

1. On the bottom of a petri dish containing nutrient agar, use a felt-tip pen to draw two intersecting lines that divide the dish into quarters. Number the quarters 1-4.
2. Using the procedure outlined in Steps 3-7 below, test the three surfaces in the variation assigned to you by your teacher.
   Variation 1. your shoulder; sink bottom; cutting board
   Variation 2. your hair; clean dish; countertop
   Variation 3. refrigerator shelf; washed fingertip; unwashed fingertip
   Variation 4. tabletop; floor; doorknob
3. Obtain a 10-cm strip of cellophane tape. Fold over about 2 cm of the tape to make a non-stick end to hold.
4. Holding the tape at the folded end, put the sticky side on one of the three surfaces named in your variation. Pull the tape from the surface, and immediately place it on the agar surface on the quarter of the dish marked number 1. Remove and discard the tape.
5. In your data table, record the source from which you took the sample and the number of the area in the dish where you put it.
6. Repeat Steps 3, 4, and 5 for each of the other two surfaces in your variation, putting each sample in a new section of the dish.
7. As a control, obtain a fourth piece of tape and touch it to the agar without letting the end that touches the agar touch any other surface, including your fingers. Repeat Step 5.
8. Incubate the petri dish at room temperature for three or four days in the place designated by your teacher.
9. Observe the petri dish daily. Describe in your data table and on the board any growths that have appeared on the agar.
10. In your data table, copy the information on the growths reported for the other variations.

Analyzing Results

1. Was the tape itself free of microorganisms?

   _____

2. Were any of the surfaces tested free of microorganisms? Which ones?

   _____

(Continued on next page)

Food Science Lab Manual
Copyright © Mehas & Rodgers

3. Which surfaces produced the most bacterial growth? Why do you think this occurred?

_____

_____

_____

4. How can you minimize the likelihood of food poisoning?

_____

_____

_____

DATA TABLE

Surface Tested	Area Number	Agar Day 1	Agar Day 2	Agar Day 3
Variation 1				
Variation 2				
Variation 3				
Variation 4				

Bacteria in Milk

EXPERIMENT 25-2

SAFETY FIRST
Review these safety guidelines before you begin this experiment.

Milk produced by a healthy cow is a completely sterile fluid. During milking, however, it passes through ducts that are normally contaminated with many types of bacteria. Unless great care is taken, these bacteria will enter the milk. If the milk is cooled immediately and kept cold, they will multiply very slowly. When milk is pasteurized, all forms of harmful bacteria are killed.

One way to test for the presence of bacteria in milk is to add the indicator called methylene blue. This blue substance becomes colorless in the absence of oxygen. Since bacteria use up the oxygen present in milk, the rate at which the methylene blue loses its color is a measure of the number of bacteria in the milk.

In this experiment, you will compare the bacteria populations in fresh raw and pasteurized milk, as well as in samples that have been kept for one week or longer.

Equipment and Materials
4 test tubes
masking tape
marking pen
10-mL graduated cylinder
raw milk (fresh and week-old)
pasteurized milk (fresh and week-old)
methylene blue solution
stirring rod
250-mL beaker
thermometer
dehydrator or incubator

Procedure

1. Label four test tubes 1-4. Add milk to the test tubes according to the following:
   Test tube 1: 10 mL of fresh raw milk
   Test tube 2: 10 mL of fresh pasteurized milk
   Test tube 3: 10 mL of week-old raw milk
   Test tube 4: 10 mL of week-old pasteurized milk
2. To each test tube, add 0.5 mL of methylene blue solution. Stir each sample to mix the indicator throughout the milk. Wash the stirring rod thoroughly after stirring each sample to avoid cross-contamination. Make note of the time that you add the solution to the test tubes.
3. Incubate the test tubes in a beaker of water heated to 37°C. Maintain the water at this temperature throughout the experiment.
4. Check the test tubes periodically over the next 24 hours. In your data table, record the time needed to completely decolorize the indicator. Milk that loses color in less than half an hour is badly contaminated. A sample that retains color for more than eight hours is of excellent quality.

(Continued on next page)

EXPERIMENT 25-2 (Continued)

Analyzing Results

1. Which sample had the fewest bacteria present? The most?

   _____
   _____

2. What does this experiment indicate about the importance of pasteurization?

   _____
   _____
   _____

3. What other steps can be taken to prevent or delay growth of bacteria in milk?

   _____
   _____
   _____
   _____

DATA TABLE

Test Tube	Time Needed to Decolorize Methylene Blue
1	
2	
3	
4	

Dehydrating Beef

EXPERIMENT 26-1

SAFETY FIRST
Review these safety guidelines before you begin this experiment.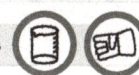

Moisture can be removed from fruits and vegetables to minimize the growth of bacteria and molds that cause them to spoil. When this technique is used with meat, the resulting product is called jerky. In this experiment you'll compare dry-cured, brine-cured, and unsalted air-dried beef. Do not eat the samples prepared.

Equipment and Materials
flank steak	250-mL beaker	marking pen	skewer
cutting board	brine solution	coarse salt	two ring stands
heavy bottle or mallet	masking tape	paper towel	two iron rings
balance			

Procedure: Day 1
1. Obtain a beef strip and lay it on a clean cutting board. Pound it with a heavy bottle or mallet until it is very thin.
2. Mass the strip and record the result in your data table.
3. Place the strip in a 250-mL beaker and add the brine solution provided by your teacher until the meat is completely covered. Label the beaker with your name and set aside until day two.

Procedure: Day 2
4. Obtain two more strips of beef and lay them on a clean cutting board. Pound them with a heavy bottle or a mallet until they are very thin.
5. Mass each of the strips and record results in your data table.
6. Place one of the strips on a clean cutting board. Sprinkle salt heavily on one side of the strip and pound it in. Turn the strip over and pound salt into the other side.
7. Remove the strip that has been soaking in the brine and pat dry with a paper towel. Hang all three strips on a shish kebab skewer. Place the ends of the skewer on two iron rings attached to ring stands. Set the iron rings high enough that the meat strips do not touch the table top. Leave until day three.

Procedure: Day 3
8. Carefully remove the strips from the skewer, determine their masses, and record in your data table. Return them to the skewer for another day.

Procedure: Day 4
9. Again, remove the strips from the skewer, determine their masses, and record the results in your data table.
10. Calculate and record the percent of mass lost, using the formula:

$$\text{percent of mass lost} = \frac{(\text{fresh mass} - \text{dried mass}) \times 100}{\text{fresh mass}}$$

11. Try breaking the jerky. Then describe its appearance and texture in your data table.

(Continued on next page)

Food Science Lab Manual
Copyright © Mehas & Rodgers

EXPERIMENT 26-1 (Continued)

Analyzing Results

1. Which method gave the toughest jerky? Which gave the most crisp?

   _____
   _____

2. What effect does salt have on the drying process?

   _____
   _____
   _____

3. Which strip lost the largest percentage of its mass during the drying period?

   _____
   _____

4. Do you think any of the strips need further drying? Why?

   _____
   _____
   _____

5. How might you determine if any of the strips still contain water?

   _____
   _____
   _____

DATA TABLE

Beef Strips	Fresh Mass	Mass Day 3	Mass Day 4	Percent Mass Lost	Appearance and Texture
Brine Cured					
Salted					
Dry Cured					

198 Food Science Lab Manual
Copyright © Mehas & Rodgers

Dehydrating Fruits and Vegetables

EXPERIMENT 26-2

SAFETY FIRST
Review these safety guidelines before you begin this experiment.

In this experiment, you will test the moisture content of various fruits and vegetables by dehydrating them and determining their loss of mass. You will assume this loss of mass is due to a loss of water.

Equipment and Materials

fruit or vegetable	sodium bisulfite solution	dehydrator and trays
paring knife	1000-mL beaker	plastic bag
paper towels	1000-mL plastic beaker	masking tape
cutting board	balance	marking pen

Procedure

1. Wash, peel, and core the fruit or vegetable provided by your teacher. Pat dry with a paper towel.
2. Place the food on a cutting board and slice into 0.3-cm slices.
3. Soak one slice of food for 5 minutes in the sodium bisulfite solution provided by your teacher. Remove the slice and rinse it lightly under cold tap water. Place it on the rack or drying tray specified by your teacher for the sodium bisulfite samples.
4. Mass the remaining food; record the value in your data table.
5. Spread the food you have massed on the rack or drying tray.
6. Place racks or trays in the dehydrator, following your teacher's directions.
7. The next day, mass the dried food and record the mass in your data table.
8. Calculate the percent of the original sample that was water. This is the percent of the original mass lost during drying. It can be determined with the following equation:

$$\text{Percent of original mass lost as water} = \frac{(\text{fresh mass} - \text{dried mass}) \times 100}{\text{fresh mass}}$$

9. Obtain your pretreated food slice. Compare its appearance to that of the rest of your dried sample. Record your observations in your data table. Expand your table on separate paper if needed.
10. Write your figures, calculations, and observations on the board. In your data table, copy this information for the other samples.
11. Place your dried food in a plastic bag and label with your name and class.
12. Store the bag in the place designated by your teacher. You will use the food in another experiment.

Analyzing Results

1. What effect did the sodium bisulfite have on the pretreated slice?

_____

_____

(Continued on next page)

2. Which food lost the most water by mass?
   _____

3. Which food lost the highest percentage of water?
   _____
   _____

4. Which fruit or vegetable originally had the highest moisture content? How did you determine this?
   _____
   _____
   _____
   _____

5. Do you think 100 percent of the water in the fresh sample was removed? Why or why not?
   _____
   _____

DATA TABLE

Food	Mass			Percent Lost as Water	Appearance of Pretreated Slice	Appearance of Untreated Food
	Original Sample	Dried Sample	Lost by Original Sample			

Reconstituting Fruits and Vegetables

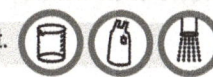
EXPERIMENT 26-3

SAFETY FIRST
Review these safety guidelines before you begin this experiment.

In this experiment, you will reconstitute the fruit or vegetable sample you dehydrated in Experiment 26-2. You will see whether it will reabsorb all the water originally lost.

Equipment and Materials
dehydrated fruit or vegetable from Experiment 26-2
1000-mL beaker
paper towels
balance
1000-mL plastic beaker

Procedure
1. In your data table, enter the mass of the dried fruit or vegetable sample from Experiment 26-2.
2. Place your dehydrated food in a 1000-mL beaker filled with water. Soak the food for 40 minutes. Drain and pat the pieces dry with a paper towel.
3. Mass the reconstituted samples. Record the reconstituted mass in your data table.
4. Calculate the amount of water absorbed by the reconstituted food. Record this value in your data table.
5. Calculate the percent of the reconstituted sample that is water. This is the same as the percent of the reconstituted mass gained during the soaking process.

$$\text{Percent of mass gained as water} = \frac{(\text{reconstituted mass} - \text{dried mass}) \times 100}{\text{reconstituted mass}}$$

6. Write your figures and calculations on the board. In your data table, copy the information on the other food samples.

Analyzing Results

1. Which fruit or vegetable absorbed the most water by mass?

2. Which fruit or vegetable gained the highest percentage of water?

(Continued on next page)

Food Science Lab Manual
Copyright © Mehas & Rodgers

EXPERIMENT 26-3 (Continued)

3. Did any fruit or vegetable restore to the original mass?
   _____
   _____

4. Would soaking the food for a longer time change the results? Why or why not?
   _____
   _____
   _____

DATA TABLE

Food	Mass			Percent of Reconstituted Mass Gained as Water
	Dried Sample	Reconstituted Sample	Gained by Reconstituted Sample	

Name _____ Date _____ Class _____

EXPERIMENT 27-1
Evaluating Canned Peas

SAFETY FIRST
Review these safety guidelines before you begin this experiment.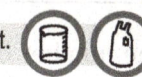

You will recall that young vegetables contain mostly sugar, which turns into starch as the vegetables age, or mature. Young peas are sweet and tender, while mature peas have a tough starchiness. Since young peas are more desirable, the most important factor in evaluating or grading peas is maturity.

There are several ways to evaluate canned peas. One method involves placing peas in a saline solution. Young tender peas float, while the mature peas sink from the density of their starch. Another way to check the maturity of peas is to observe the liquid, or brine, in which the peas are packed. The starch in mature peas dissolves into the brine, creating a cloudy effect. Finally, the skin of mature peas is often split and broken, while young peas are apt to have smooth, unbroken skins. This experiment lets you use all three methods to evaluate various brands of canned peas.

Equipment and Materials
canned peas
can opener
200 mL saline solution
100-mL graduated cylinder
250-mL beakers
slotted spoon
paper towel
100-mL beaker
masking tape
marking pen

Procedure
1. Count 50 peas from the source indicated by your teacher.
2. Pour 200 mL of the saline solution provided by your teacher into a 250-mL beaker.
3. Add the peas to the saline solution, and observe for 30-60 seconds. Count how many peas sink to the bottom. If nearly all the peas sink, count how many remain floating and subtract from 50. Record this information in your data table.
4. Remove the peas from the saline solution, and place them on a paper towel. Count how many peas in your sample have broken skins. Record this information in your data table.
5. Place 50 mL of pea brine in a 100-mL beaker, label it with the brand name, and place in the area designated by your teacher. Note the appearance of the brine, compare it to the other brands, and record the information in your data table.
6. Obtain unit cost information for your brand of peas from your teacher, and write it in your data table.
7. Write your information on the board. In your data table, copy the information about the other brands of peas.

Analyzing Results
1. Which brand of peas had the largest number of peas that sank? The smallest number?

_____

_____

(Continued on next page)

Food Science Lab Manual
Copyright © Mehas & Rodgers

2. Which brand of peas had the largest number of peas with split skins? The smallest number?

_____

_____

3. Was there any relationship between the number of peas that sank and the number that had broken skins? Explain.

_____

_____

_____

4. Was there any relationship between the number of peas that sank and the cloudiness of the brine from which they came? Explain.

_____

_____

_____

_____

5. Which brand of peas seemed to be of the highest quality?

_____

6. Were the peas with the highest unit cost the ones of the highest quality?

DATA TABLE

Brand of Peas	Number That Sank	Number with Broken Skins	Appearance of Brine	Unit Cost

(Continued on next page.)

Name _____ Date _____ Class _____

Environment and Bacteria

EXPERIMENT 27-2

SAFETY FIRST
Review these safety guidelines before you begin this experiment.

A number of factors determine whether a given environment will promote the growth of microorganisms. This experiment will illustrate some of the factors that affect bacterial growth.

Equipment and Materials

chicken broth	6 beakers, 50-mL	sugar	stirring rod
250-mL beaker	beaker tongs	salt	tweezers
safety goggles	masking tape	water	microscope and slide
saucepan	marking pen	lemon juice	

Procedure

1. Place 200 mL of chicken broth in a 250-mL beaker.
2. Heat the broth-filled beaker on a medium-high setting. Boil the broth for 5 minutes. Wear safety goggles during the heating process. Remove the broth from the heat using beaker tongs, and cool for at least 5 minutes or until the beaker is cool enough to handle safely.
3. Fill a large saucepan with tap water. Bring the water to a boil. Wear safety goggles while the water is boiling.
4. Place six empty 50-mL beakers in the boiling water for 5 minutes to sterilize. Remove each beaker with tongs, drain, and cool.
5. Fill each of the beakers half full of chicken broth.
6. Use masking tape to label the beakers A, B, C, D, E, and F. Also label with your name and class.
7. Add the following substances to the specified beakers and stir. Use a clean stirring rod in each beaker.
   Beaker A: 5 mL sugar
   Beaker B: 2.5 mL salt
   Beaker C: 5 mL salt
   Beaker D: 5 mL water
   Beaker E: 5 mL lemon juice
   Beaker F: nothing
8. Store the beakers per teacher instructions.
9. On the sixth day, observe each sample for color, general appearance, and odor. *Do not taste the broth.* Record your observations.
10. If mold has appeared on your broth, use tweezers to transfer a sample of it from the beaker to a microscope slide. Try not to crush the mold as you transfer it. Examine it under a microscope. Include drawings of the mold in your lab report.

Analyzing Results

1. Which sample differed most from the others? In what ways?

_____

_____

(Continued on next page)

Food Science Lab Manual
Copyright © Mehas & Rodgers

2. Which samples were most similar in their properties? In what ways?

_____

_____

3. Which beakers contained mold? Why do you suppose mold grew in those beakers and not the others?

_____

_____

_____

4. How do you think your results would differ if you had refrigerated the samples?

_____

_____

DATA TABLE

Beaker	Color	Appearance	Odor
A			
B			
C			
D			
E			
F			

206
Food Science Lab Manual
Copyright © Mehas & Rodgers

Name _____ Date _____ Class _____

Orange Juice Comparison

EXPERIMENT 28-1

SAFETY FIRST
Review these safety guidelines before you begin this experiment.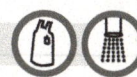

The method used to preserve a food can affect the properties and quality of the food. In this experiment, you will use your knowledge of sensory evaluation to compare samples of fresh, frozen, freeze-dried, aseptically processed, and pouch-canned orange juices.

Equipment and Materials
5 paper cups, 28-mL
samples of orange juice: fresh squeezed; reconstituted frozen; reconstituted freeze-dried; pouch canned; and aseptically canned
masking tape
marking pen

Procedure

1. Compare the samples provided by your teacher on color, mouthfeel, and taste. Enter the information in your data table.

2. Your teacher will provide information on unit cost and the preservation method of each sample. Enter the information in your data table.

Analyzing Results

1. Which sample looked most like fresh orange juice?
   _____

2. Which sample "felt" most like fresh orange juice?
   _____

3. Which sample had the best taste?
   _____

4. Which juice would you rank the highest overall?
   _____

(Continued on next page)

Food Science Lab Manual
Copyright © Mehas & Rodgers

EXPERIMENT 28-1 (Continued)

5. How does the juice that you ranked highest compare to the other samples in unit cost?

   _____

   _____

   _____

6. Which juice would you buy to drink regularly? Why?

   _____

   _____

   _____

7. Which juice would you take camping? Why?

   _____

   _____

   _____

DATA TABLE

Sample	Color	Mouthfeel	Taste	Unit Cost	Preservation Method